Fair Shakes: The Health Care Compensation Handbook

American Society for Hospital Personnel Administration
of the American Hospital Association

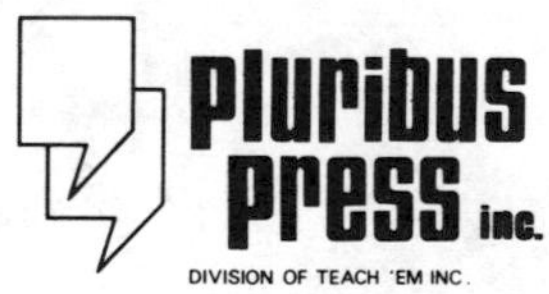

160 East Illinois Street
Chicago, IL 60611

Library of Congress Catalog Card Number

84-60859

Fair Shakes: The Health Care Compensation Handbook

International Standard Book Number
0-931028-52-3

Published in conjunction with Pluribus Press, Inc.,
160 E. Illinois St., Chicago, IL 60611.

MANUAL FOR
DEVELOPING AN EMPLOYEE COMPENSATION PROGRAM

MANUAL TOPICS

PREFACE

In a continuing effort to enhance the knowledge and skills of human resources professionals, The American Society for Hospital Personnel Administration (ASHPA) has developed this manual on job evaluation and compensation. The manual is designed to present the new compensation specialists with tools for establishing or revising their organizations' comprehensive job evaluation and compensation program. It will also provide the human resources management department with a ready reference since it contains a number of job descriptions for key hospital positions.

ASHPA wishes to thank a number of individuals who have been instrumental in developing this important new manual.

We would like to thank Compensation Systems, Inc., of Bannockburn, IL, for their development of the original manuscript. Additional work on the book was done by Michael Maciekowich, former manager of compensation and benefits with the AHA Division of Employee Relations, and currently compensation consultant with Compensation Systems, Inc. We also want to thank Jeff Rogers, Director of Human Resources, St. Joseph Hospital, Phoenix, for his expert review of the manuscript. Several staff from the AHA Office of Human Resources were instrumental in writing and producing the book, including Kevin F. Hickey, Director; Emmett L. Kennedy, Staff Specialist; Barbara Bloom Kreml, Senior Staff Specialist; and V. Brandon Melton, Manager.

INTRODUCTION

The 1970's brought to the health care industry increased complexity in the design and development of compensations programs. The individuals responsible for developing, administering and maintaining the institution's pay programs must become increasingly concerned with the following:

* Complying with various laws, regulations and executive orders from local, state, and federal agencies.
* Coping with fluctuations in the economy, such as reduced resources resulting from changes in the reimbursement system.
* Responding to increased employee awareness and concern for internal and external equity.
* Assuring effective spending of payroll dollars which comprise 50% or more of the hospital's operating budget.
* Dealing with shortages of qualified health care personnel.

These and other continuing challenges underscore the need to have a formal, logical, equitable, and defensible system of employee compensation in health care institutions.

All health care facilities-- hospitals, health maintenance organizations, nursing homes, clinics, ambulatory care centers-- whether proprietary, non-profit or governmental, have similar objectives and goals in the design of their compensation programs. These objectives are:

* to attract qualified employees
* to retain those employees
* to motivate the employee to perform the duties and tasks of the job in the most effective manner

In arriving at a specific amount of money to pay for a given job or for a given employee, the hospital must take into account both external and internal factors. External factors include market factors and specific laws and government regulations. Internal factors are job criteria, the management's pay philosophy, style of management, and its ability to pay the individual employee according to experience, seniority, and performance.

In cases where a facility has limited financial resources, the market rate for jobs must be seriously considered. In order to achieve the three specified objectives of a compensation program previously identified, the hospital cannot, for very long, pay significantly below the market rate, as qualified employees will seek employment elsewhere at the higher market rate.* Alternatively, the hospital cannot consistently pay at levels significantly above the market rate for employees, because the hospital's competitive position will erode in the long run. If the hospital's wage costs are higher than its competition's without offsetting greater productivity, the unit labor costs will escalate.

The hospital's internal assessment of the worth of a job may sometimes conflict with the labor market price. These conflicts tend to operate over time as the forces of supply and demand operate in the external market. The pay system should be flexible enough to respond effectively to both market forces and internal considerations.

The hospital must make a number of decisions in trying to achieve the goals of the compensation program. These dec-

---

* For clarity, the term "hospital" is used in referring to the employer. However, the system described in this manual is applicable to any health facility as indicated in the text.

isions include what pay philosophy the hospital desires to adopt and practice, recognizing that certain limitations have been established by society through various laws such as the Fair Labor Standards Act, Equal Employment Opportunity Act and Equal Pay Act. These statutory considerations will be outlined and addressed in more detail in the following section of this manual.

It should be recognized that there are a number of methods to accomplish an organization's pay program goals and objectives. Some hospitals tend to solve the question of what to pay their employees by directly relating salaries to the competitive marketplace, disregarding internal considerations. Other hospitals administer more formal systems of evaluating and pricing jobs. Techniques that have been developed over the past several decades measure specifically identified compensable factors and the extent to which they are present in each job. These systems invariably incorporate competitive considerations into the overall program.

Benefit levels, such as life insurance, social security, pension plans, and in some cases, shift differentials, tie in directly as a percentage of base salary. Therefore, base salary is the core around which all elements of cash and non-cash compensation revolve. This means that as base salary increases, so does related non-cash compensation. The following diagram illustrates this point:

TOTAL COMPENSATION

Vacation
Soc. Secur-ity
Shft Diff
BASE SAL.
Life Ins.
Pension

TOTAL COMPENSATION

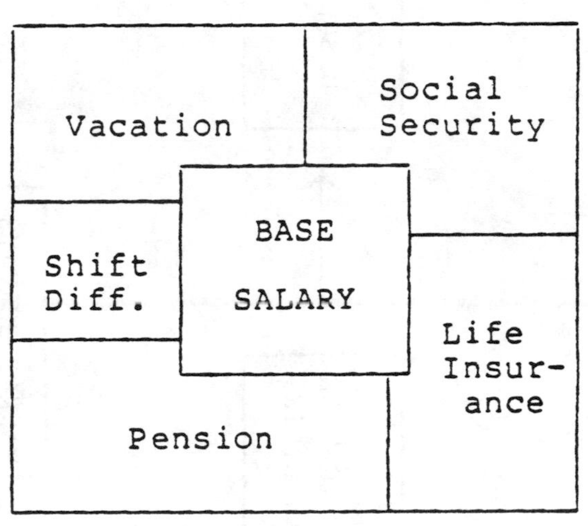

This manual has been written to assist hospitals in the design of a compensation program for all positions up to and including department heads. The manual is a "hands-on" reference for those who want to develop or refresh their knowledge of the concepts, techniques, and processes which are basic to a good compensation program. Each section of the manual addresses a specific phase in the development of a sound compensation program.

THE TOTAL COMPENSATION PROCESS

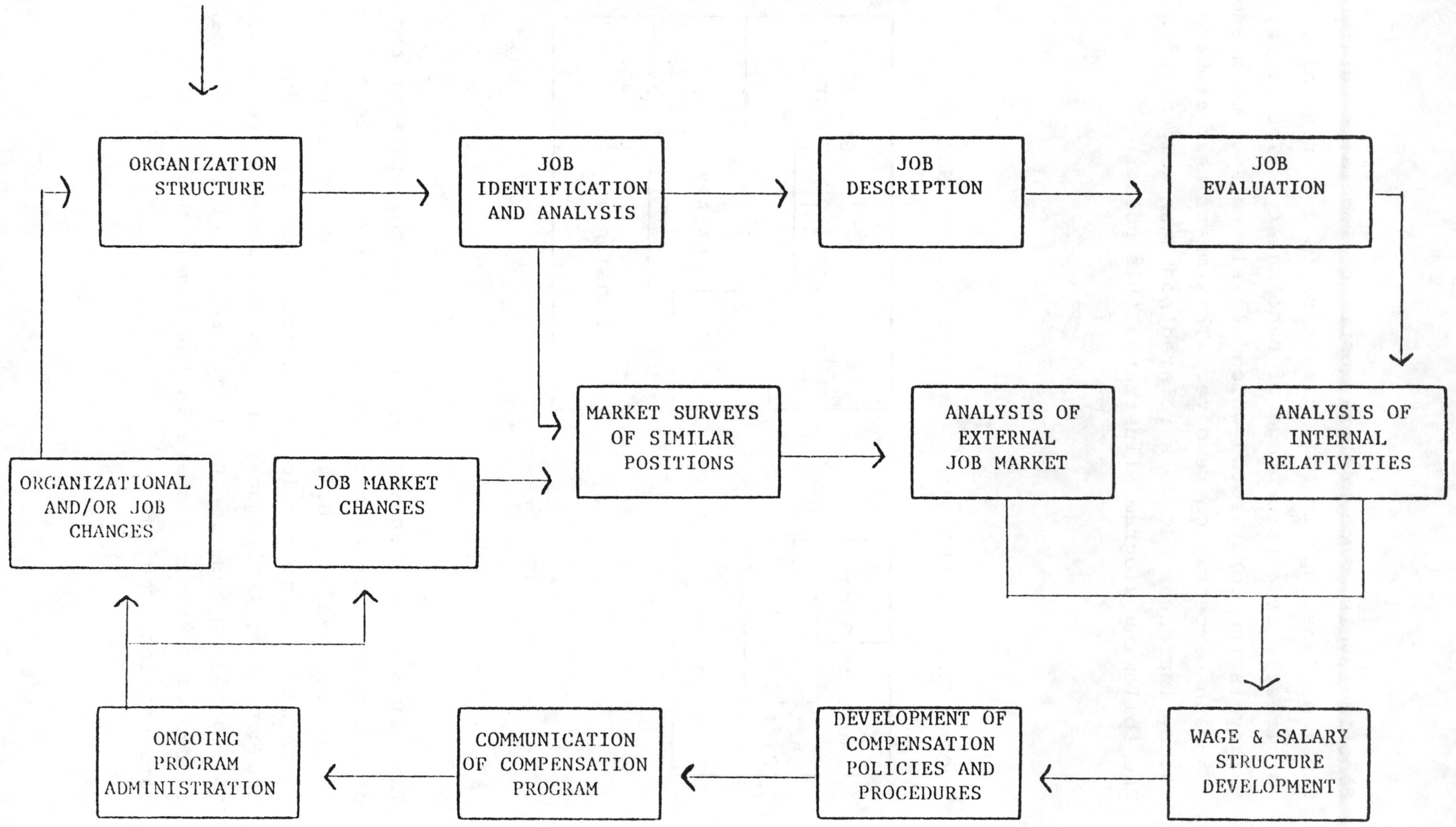

ORGANIZATION STRUCTURE

JOB IDENTIFICATION AND ANALYSIS

JOB DESCRIPTION

JOB EVALUATION

MARKET SURVEYS OF SIMILAR POSITIONS

ANALYSIS OF EXTERNAL JOB MARKET

ANALYSIS OF INTERNAL RELATIVITIES

ORGANIZATIONAL AND/OR JOB CHANGES

JOB MARKET CHANGES

WAGE & SALARY STRUCTURE DEVELOPMENT

DEVELOPMENT OF COMPENSATION POLICIES AND PROCEDURES

COMMUNICATION OF COMPENSATION PROGRAM

ONGOING PROGRAM ADMINISTRATION

SECTION I

STATUTORY CONSIDERATIONS

STATUTORY CONSIDERATIONS

Over the last 50 years, the government has become increasingly involved in the procedures and operations of organizations. One of the areas where government activity recently has been most visible has been in the development of regulations and guidelines concerning the organization's treatment of its employees. As a result, organizations are forced to respond to local, state, and federal laws and agencies such as the Equal Opportunity Commission and the Wage and Hour Division of the Department of Labor. For this reason, current statutes and government guidelines must be considered in the development and administration of a compensation program.

While certain state laws may differ slightly from others, the predominant impact is brought about by the following Statutes:

- Fair Labor Standards Act

- Equal Employment Opportunity Commission (Title VII of the Civil Rights Act)

- Equal Pay Act

FAIR LABOR STANDARDS ACT OF 1938

The Fair Labor Standards Act is also referred to as the Wage and Hour Law. As amended in 1966 and 1974, the FLSA covers two important issues for the hospital compensation administrator: 1) minimum-wage, and 2) overtime, as these provisions apply to hospital employees.

Minimum Wage

The Act requires that all non-exempt employees be paid at hourly rates at least equal to the current minimum wage level, as set by Congress. Historically, this wage has been annually revised and adjusted up, effective January 1 of each year.

The Act also requires uniform allowances for employees who are required to wear uniforms and who are paid minimum wage, plus 7 to 8 cents.

Overtime Pay Requirements

The overtime provisions require payment of one and one-half times the employee's regular rate of pay to all non-exempt employees for hours worked above eight hours per shift or in excess of 80 hours during the 14 day period, whichever is greater, and/or a 40-hour week.

Hospitals may also elect to pay employees on the basis of eight hours in a shift or in excess of 80 hours during the 14 day work period provided this agreement is made at the time of employment. This option provides additional flexibility for scheduling workers on a 24-hour basis. Again, all non-exempt employees who work more than eight hours or more than 80 hours in a consecutive two-week period must receive one and one-half times their regular rate of pay for each additional hour worked. Regular rate of pay is defined as:

$$\frac{\text{Total compensation in work week, minus pay for time not worked, plus unrestricted call wages}}{\text{Divided by hours worked (including unrestricted call hours)}}$$

The law requires that records of hours worked in increments of one-tenth of an hour be maintained for all non-exempt employees:

Determination of Exempt or Non-Exempt Status

Exemption from provisions of the Act are possible, if jobs meet certain specific tests to classify them as exempt. The following categories of hospital employees are exempt by the FLSA law:

- Executive
- Administrative
- Professional
- Outside Sales

1. Executive Employee Exemption

A. Qualifying Tests

An employee is exempt from the overtime provisions of the Act if duties and responsibilities meet all six of the executive qualifying tests.

- If the primary duty of the position is management of the hospital, one of its departments, or sub-units.

- If the position directs the work of two or more employees.

- If the position has the authority to hire or fire other employees, or to make recommendations that will be given particular weight in the hiring, firing, and the advancement, promotion or other change of status of other employees.

- If the position requires regular exercise of discretionary powers.

- If the position does not devote more than 40% of the hours worked in the work week to non-exempt work.

- If the individual receives pay on a salary basis at a rate of not less than $155 per week ($671.67 per month).

B. <u>Special Proviso Tests</u>

An employee may be considered exempt if duties and responsibilities meet Special Proviso Test A and B.

TEST A: The employee is paid a salary of $250.00 per week ($1,083.33 per month), or more, effective April 1, 1975, AND,

TEST B: The employee meets the first two executive status qualifying tests above. (It is not necessary to apply the other executive status qualifying tests above when applying the Special Proviso Tests.)

ADMINISTRATIVE EMPLOYEE EXEMPTION

A. Qualifying Tests

An employee is exempt from the overtime provisions of the Act if duties and responsibilities meet all five of the administrative qualifying tests below:

- 1. If the employee is performing office or non-manual work directly related to management policies or the general business operations of the employer/patients; OR,

  2. If the employee's primary duty is performing work directly related to academic instruction or training in an educational institution, or the academic administration or operation of an educational departmental subdivision or larger unit.

- If the employee customarily and regularly exercises discretion and independent judgment.

- 1. If the employee regularly and directly assists an executive or administrative exempt employee; OR,

2. If the employee works under only general supervision along specialized or technical lines which require special training, experience or knowledge; OR,

3. If the employee executes special assignments or tasks under only general supervision.

- If the employee does not devote more than 40% of the hours worked in a work week to activities which are not directly and closely related to those in the above tests.

NOTE: Non-exempt work is typically work that is standardized; or involving routine mental, manual or physical processes; or requiring only general manual or intellectual ability; and not directly and closely related to exempt duties and responsibilities, as outlined.

- 1. If the same salary test as for the Executive Exemption applies to the employee--$155.00 per week ($671.67 per month), or more, effective April 1, 1975; OR,

  2. Salary for academic administrative personnel--If the salary of the employee is at least equal to the entrance salaries for teachers in the same educational institution.

B. Special Proviso Tests

An employee may be considered exempt if duties and responsibilities meet Special Proviso Tests A and B.

TEST A: If the employee is paid a salary of $250.00 per week ($1,083.33 per month), or more, effective April 1, 1975; AND,

TEST B: If the employee meets the first two administrative status qualifying tests above. (It is not necessary to apply the remaining qualifying tests above when applying the Special Proviso Tests.)

PROFESSIONAL EMPLOYEE EXEMPTION

A. Qualifying Tests

An employee is exempt from the overtime provisions of the Act if his duties and responsibilities meet all five of the qualifying tests below:

- 1. If the position's primary duty is performing work requiring knowledge of an advanced type in a field of science or learning customarily acquired by a prolonged course of specialized intellectual instruction and study; OR,

2. If the position's primary duty is performing work that is original and creative in character in a recognized field of scientific endeavor, requiring invention, imagination or talent to achieve satisfactory results; OR,

3. If the position's primary duty is imparting knowledge through teaching, tutoring, instruction or lecturing as a recognized or certified teacher.

- Performance in the job requires the consistent exercise of discretion and judgment.

- If the employee performs work predominantly intellectual and varied in character with an output or result that cannot be standardized in terms of time.

- If at least 80% of the employee's hours of work in the work week are an essential part of and necessarily incident to the above tests (i.e., the employee performs non-exempt work no more than 20% of his time).

<u>NOTE</u>: Non-exempt work is typically work that is standardized; or involving routine mental, manual or physical processes; or requiring general manual or intellectual ability; <u>and is not an essential part of and necessarily incident to exempt duties and responsibilities, as outlined</u>.

- 1. If the employee's salary or fee is $170.00 per week ($736.67 per month), or more, effective April 1, 1975; OR,

  2. If the employee holds a valid license or certificate permitting the practice of law or medicine, or any of their branches, and the employee is actually engaged in such practice; OR,

3. If the employee holds the requisite academic degree for the general practice of medicine and is engaged in an intern or resident capacity, pursuant to the practice of medicine or any of its branches; OR,

4. If the employee is employed and engaged as a recognized or certified teacher.

B. Special Proviso Tests

An employee may be considered exempt if his duties and responsibilities meet Special Proviso Tests A and B.

TEST A: If the employee is paid a salary or fee of $250.00 per week ($1,083.33 per month), or more, effective April 1, 1975; AND,

TEST B: If the employee meets the first two professional status qualifying tests above. (It is not necessary to apply the remaining qualifying tests above when applying the Special Proviso Tests.)

OUTSIDE SALES REPRESENTATIVE EXEMPTION

Though this exemption does not generally apply to hospital positions, briefly, the tests are as follows:

A. Qualifying Tests

An employee is exempt from the overtime provisions of the Act if duties and responsibilities meet both of the Outside Sales Representative qualifying tests:

- If the employee is customarily and regularly engaged away from the employer's place (or places) of business and employed for the purpose of:

   1. Making sales, OR,

   2. Obtaining orders or contracts for services or for the use of facilities.

- If the employee does not perform work other than that described in the above test which exceeds 20% of the hours worked in the work week by non-exempt employees. (The 20% is computed on the basis of the hours worked by non-exempt employees of the employer who perform the kind of non-exempt work performed by the outside sales representative-- <u>except</u> -- work performed incidental to and in conjunction with the employee's own outside sales or solicitations shall not be regarded as non-exempt work.)

  <u>NOTE</u>: Non-exempt work is typically work that is standardized; or involving routine mental, manual or physical processes; or requiring only general manual or intellectual ability; <u>and not incidental to and in conjunction with exempt duties and responsibilities, as outlined</u>.

<u>COMBINATION EXEMPTION</u>

Combination exemptions (tacking of exempt work under one section of the regulation to exempt work of another) are permissible under the Fair Labor Standards

Act. However, the employee must meet the stricter of the requirements on salary and non-exempt work, regardless of which exempt function occupies most of his time.

	Executive	Administrative	Professional
Salary (Effective April 1, 1975)	$155.00/wk $671.67/mo	$155.00/wk $671.67/mo	$170.00/wk $736.67/mo
Percentage of non-exempt work	40%	40%	20%

The following combination exemptions exist:

Combination Possibilities	Salary	Percentage of Non-exempt work
Executive Administrative	$155.00/wk $671.67/mo	20%
Executive Professional	$170.00/wk $736.67/mo	20%
Administrative Professional	$170.00/wk $736.67/mo	20%

In summary, determination of FLSA status is based on the job duties and responsibilities. As a result, all employees with the same job title should have the same FLSA status. In gray areas where exempt status is uncertain, it is recommended that the position be classified as non-exempt.

EQUAL EMPLOYMENT OPPORTUNITY COMMISSION

(TITLE VII OF THE CIVIL RIGHTS ACT)

With respect to a compensation program, the EEOC establishes criteria upon which minimum job qualifications may be established. Simply stated:

1. Job qualifications should be job-related and required for an individual to perform the minimum standards of the job.

2. Where necessary, an employer may be called upon to demonstrate that such requirements are necessary.

3. Under certain conditions, required qualifications may be waived.

Title VII of the Civil Rights Act does not allow for any job requirement which disqualifies individuals based on race, color, religion, sex, national origin, or age. However, an exception can be made in terms of these factors if it is shown that they are "bona fide occupational qualifications (BFOQ)." The claim that any one of these factors is a bona fide occupational qualification is one which must be made carefully. The EEOC has taken a strict view in this area and requires complete substantiation.

EQUAL PAY ACT

The Equal Pay Act is a federal act which stipulates that there may be no differentiation in pay for equal work on the basis of sex.

While there may be no disagreement with the need and the validity of this act, several areas of discussion have arisen, chiefly concerned with:

1. The definition of what constitutes equal work.

2. The demonstration of differerces in effort between incumbents both classified in the same job.

Federal regulations classify the generic basis or classification upon which equal work may be judged. These include skill, responsibility, effort (mental and physical) and working conditions.

The Equal Pay Act does allow for pay differentials if the rates are based on a merit system, a productivity standard, seniority, or any basis other than sex. Employees hired on a temporary basis may be paid at a rate lower than permanent employees.

However, the issue of equal pay for equal work has been expanded in recent years to include equal pay for comparable work.

COMPARABLE WORTH

During the past five years, there has been much debate as to whether the term "equal work" implies jobs which are exactly the same, or jobs which are different but of comparable worth to the employer. With the idea of comparable worth, the nature of the jobs does not need to be related in any way. Comparable worth means the value of the work is of comparable or similar value to the employer, and thus payment for the work should be the same. This doctrine is based on the idea that certain professions and positions traditionally have been undervalued, and underpaid, because they primarily have been held by women. Proponents of this doctrine claim that because positions have similar value but are paid at different levels, discrimination based on sex exists.

Sex discrimination cases are covered under the Equal Pay Act and Title VII of the Civil Rights Act, although those acts do not consider the idea of comparable worth. An amendment to Title VII, the Bennett Amendment, allows for the filing of such suits.

This amendment states that where there is conflict between the Equal Pay Act and Title VII, the Equal Pay Act will rule. However, the primary issue remains whether "comparable worth" should be equated with "equal worth" as defined by law. To date, most court cases have been decided on the basis of whether the Equal Pay Act or Title VII was violated. Such cases have established precedents by which many compensation practices, such as job evaluations and salary surveys, have been questioned, thus placing pressure on employees in terms of ensuring fairness in pay programs.

Due to the uncertainty of the issues involved, as well as the future actions by Congress and the courts, employers should take a careful look at their current pay policies and the possibility of discrimination claims. Employers should review and "audit" their compensation programs on an ongoing basis in terms of discrimination. Specifically, employers should:

* Review the process by which pay rates are set
* Review all exceptions to current pay practice
* Review the evaluation of like or similar positions across job family lines (jobs grouped together by markets or other similarities)
* Develop a strong internal auditing system in regard to pay practices

EXECUTIVE ORDER 11246

The Executive Order is similar to Title VII in that it prohibits employment discrimination based on race, national origin, color, creed, religion and sex. It is enforced by the Office of Federal Contract Compliance Programs of the Department of Labor and applies to employers who do business with the federal government by contracts exceeding $10,000 annually. The Order provides for the development of written affirmative action programs (AAP's) by employers of at least 50 persons who also have contracts exceeding $50,000. Review of AAP's is carried out through on-site audits of employment or personnel records. Such audits include a study of the payroll records and compensation policies with an intention of finding and obtaining back wages for any discriminatory practices.

AGE DISCRIMINATION IN EMPLOYMENT ACT

The ADEA is a federal statute prohibiting the use of age as a factor in making employment related decisions. It applies to all employees or job applicants between the ages of 40 and 70,* and was enacted with the purpose of preventing the involuntary retirement of otherwise qualified workers. Its scope also encompasses such issues as hiring, job assignment, training, transfer, wages, benefits (health, welfare and pension), performance evaluation, layoff and discharge.

Any employee compensation program designer and/or administrator must not only be aware of the ADEA's scope, but must be prepared to eliminate any references to or consideration of age (either intentional or inadvertent) from wage planning when such considerations are in violation of the law. The standard exceptions to the prohibition of age as a factor occur when:

1. age is a bona fide occupational qualification;
2. decisions are based on the operation of a bona fide seniority system; and
3. the decision to enforce involuntary retirement is taken with respect to a bona fide senior executive who has an employer provided pension, profit sharing, savings and/or deferred compensation plan equalling at least an annual retirement income of $27,000.

---

* Several states have enacted age discrimination laws which express no upper limitation on the age of persons who may seek the protection of the law in order to obtain or preserve jobs.

This statute is enforced in accordance with FLSA powers, remedies and procedures by the EEOC, which may issue related regulations having the force of law. Employees may file individual lawsuits to obtain back pay and other damages from employers. The EEOC may also initiate legal actions. Such trials may be brought before a jury and the courts are empowered to award double damages where it is determined that an employer willfully violated the law.

Vocational Rehabilitation Act, and Vietnam Era Veterans Readjustment Assistance Act

By these statutes discrimination in employment against the handicapped and eligible veterans is prohibited. They are applicable to employers doing business with the federal government or receiving federal financial assistance.

Knowledge of these federal statutes are important to the salary and wage administrator insofar as they require job accommodation or modification to permit the employment of disabled veterans and handicapped persons. Although the related regulations recognize the impact on productivity that may be caused by job simplification they absolutely prohibit reductions in the wages of such persons on account of job modifications or the employee's receipt of disability income from outside sources.

COST OF LIVING INCREASES

Many organizations inside and outside the health care industry give a cost of living adjustment (COLA) to all employees on a periodic basis. Frequently, a standard formula is developed, giving a percentage of the cost of living indicator increase as a COLA general increase. (A common example of a policy is to give a 3% COLA, or general increase, for every 5% in the local cost of living indicator.)

Whether or not to give COLAs is a matter for a hospital management to decide. However, there are two important hazards to avoid in adopting such a policy.

1. Cost of living indicators do not accurately reflect the actual inflation experienced by most employees; for example, it assumes that all departments are refinanced on a monthly basis of current interest rates.

2. The administration of COLAs may cause hospital salaries to become significantly out of line with the external pay levels, which historically have not increased as rapidly as cost of living indicators, forcing the hospital to pay higher rates than the market requires.

3. COLAs, if granted, should be given to each employee category. Otherwise, the COLA would reduce the traditional differentials between those receiving the adjustment and those who do not (i.e., supervisors and department heads vis a vis the rank and file employees). This process is called salary compression.

STATEMENT OF POLICY

A compensation program will be ineffective unless it has the support of hospital senior management and the governing body. Before designing and implementing a salary and wage program, the goals of the program should be clearly defined and in line with the general management philosophies of the institution. Some hospital wish to recognize individual performance through merit programs, and others to focus on job tenure. Top hospital management and the governing body should jointly issue a statement of the policies and goals of the hospital compensation program.

Common statements of policy read like the following, as issued by top management, using AHA Community Hospital as an example:

Compensation Policy

It is the policy of Community Hospital and Medical Center to maintain wage and salary administration programs and procedures which encourage and reward superior performance and are competitive with our relevant job market competition. It is also the policy of Community to administer the wage and salary programs without regard to race, creed, color, religion, national origin, sex, handicap, or any other non-compensable factor.

The wage and salary administration program has been adopted to meet the following objectives:

- Attract and retain a highly qualified work force.
- Stimulate superior performance by reflecting, in the compensation treatment, individual differences in performance.
- Provide for equitable compensation in relation to duties, responsibilities, and relevant job market competition.
- Allow delegation of compensation administration to each manager who is responsible for evaluating others' performance.
- Provide a framework for systematically updating levels of pay and accommodating new positions.

SECTION II

INTERNAL EQUITY

A. What Is Internal Equity?

Throughout this manual the term internal equity is used frequently. A basic premise is that it's a good thing to achieve and a great deal of effort is put into this section to describe how this can be accomplished. But, what does it mean? Very simply, internal equity, as it relates to compensation, is fair pay treatment of one job versus another within an organization based on a clear rationale. This section will deal with the basic elements that go into the design of an internally equitable wage administration system and will present a model to which this approach should be applied.

B. <u>Job Identification and Documentation</u>

A basic requirement for establishing internal equity among the hospital jobs is a thorough understanding of both the exact number and identification, or title, of all the different positions that currently exist. This means that a significant amount of job facts must be gathered, analyzed and recorded in an organized format for each distinct position.

This process of gathering current job documentation is an extremely worthwhile endeavor as this information can be used for a number of purposes. For example, job documentation will:

- Assist in recruiting and interviewing potential employees.

- Assist in structuring departments to eliminate overlap or gaps in responsibilities. It is not uncommon that this process will significantly reduce the number of job titles in use because it provides a means by which jobs with similar content may be grouped together and identified as one job.

- Provide a basis for measuring changes in job content. Job responsibilities and duties frequently change over time. By providing a written record of a job at a particular time, it becomes possible to measure the signficance of the change and, if appropriate, to document and justify a change in pay.

- Assist in communications between the employee and supervisor. The job documentation process should involve those individuals most knowledgeable about the position-- namely the persons performing the job and the immediate supervisor. It should be understood and agreed to by both parties. This documentation , therefore, becomes an important element in setting performance standards, conducting performance appraisals and counseling.

- Assist in conducting or analyzing wage and salary surveys. As will be discussed later in Section III, accurate job documentation assists in making meaningful comparisons on job content and in determining the appropriate nature of external market data.

For purposes of compensation administration, one of the most important uses of the job description is that it provides management and others with a clear understanding of the level of the job, its working relationships, and its skill and work requirements in relation to other jobs in the hospital. In other words, it provides a record of duties and responsibilities for comparison to other jobs and, therefore, assists management in the job evaluation process to establish internal pay equity.

1. Job Documentation and Collection Techniques

There are a number of different techniques which have been used in the collection of job information. As has been stated, the best of these always includes participation of both the incumbent and the immediate supervisor.

Individual Interview - This method involves recording information from the supervisor and the incumbent on a standardized form. The interview is usually conducted by a personnel representative and is considered to be one of the most reliable methods to obtain detailed and accurate information. The disadvantage, however, is that this method may be slow and time-consuming, often making it impractical within the hospital.

Observation Interview - This method is similar to the individual interview except the information is gathered on the work site while the incumbent performs the job tasks. This method does not take away from the job and works well for jobs with observable manual activity. Like the individual interview, however, the collection process may be slow, time-consuming, and costly.

Diary or Work Log Method - In this technique, the incumbent is asked to keep a record of activities as they are performed. This method usually produces precise information about the duties and time spent on such activities and the sequence of events.

Questionnaire - This method involves the completion of a survey instrument regarding specific facts on each position. Employers are asked to complete the form independently and to describe the job responsibilities in their own words. This technique works well in a hospital setting where jobs are diversified, a majority of employees can express themselves in writing, and the population may be relatively large. In the case of incomplete or difficult to interpret responses, clarification can be made by conducting follow-up individual or observation interviews.

Exhibit II-1A is a sample of a job questionnaire, which when completed by employees, will provide information concerning their understanding of their:

- Job title.
- Basic purpose of the job.
- Principal or typical duties.
- Percentage of time engaged in typical duties.
- Background information related to education, experience and personal qualities.
- Supervision of others.
- Work environment including work schedules and hazards.
- Work materials and equipment.

The questionnaire establishes a basis for determining the number of jobs required and their titles, in that similiar questionnaires may be grouped together and classified as one job.

The questionnaire will provide the data necessary to analyze jobs by content. Each questionnaire should be reviewed by the immediate supervisor to assure that it is correct and complete. Any areas of disagreement concerning the job questionnaire should be clarified during the review process.

In addition, it is necessary that the questionnaire be designed to provide information relating to the compensable factors (described later) that will be examined in the job evaluation process. As will be seen, this _sample_ job questionnaire has been specifically designed to correspond to the job evaluation plan presented later in this Section.

2. Job Descriptions

Although the job questionnaire or other job documentation collection techniques provide the initial facts from each incumbent to analyze for job content, a formal job description is ususally prepared to assure that all jobs are summarized and presented in a uniform manner.

The formal job description will vary depending upon its purpose but basically it should include:

- Job title or identification.
- Basic job purpose.
- Clarification on reporting relationships or level of authority exercised.
- Description of typical scope of action.
- Description of representative duties performed.
- Description of working conditions.

In general, the format should be kept simple. The description should be short and concise and written in a non-technical and direct style. Its purpose is to describe the job, not the employee. It should not be a procedural instruction or "how to" list but rather a a description of responsibilities. Finally, it should not reflect value judgments but rather be factual, specific and definitive. As in the case of the job questionnaire, it should relate the job data to the compensable factors of the job evaluation plan in a direct manner. This helps to reduce the judgmental influence as much as possible. Samples of typical job descriptions found in most health care institutions can be found in Appendix A.

3. Generic Hospital Job Descriptions

For the purposes of this manual, generic hospital job descriptions have been developed and can be found in Appendix A. These generic descriptions are included in this manual to provide a:

- Model of job description that hospitals can use to develop descriptions tailored to their own needs.

- Sample job descriptions to use in learning the application of the job evaluation plan.

C. Job Evaluation

The next major component in establishing internal equity is the job evaluation process. Job evaluation is a method which is both logical and systematic, used to determine the relative value of one job in comparison to others in an organization--in this case, the hospital setting.

The evaluation process forms the basis or rationale for establishing equitable relationships between jobs, and provides the means by which the value of dissimilar positions can be compared on an equitable and consistent basis.

It is through the evaluation process that groupings of substantially equivalent jobs can be achieved; it provides, therefore, a foundation for fair and equitable internal pay treatment. The word "internal" must be emphasized at this point because the job evaluation process that will be presented in this manual is designed to look at positions within the same hospital. It does not address the external job market pay levels which will be discussed in Section III. Experience indicates that this is the most logical approach, in that frequently, it is the internal inequities which cause the most dissatisfaction among employees. If through job evaluation these inequities can be identified and resolved in a logical and explainable fashion, external job market factors can be applied later when developing the actual salary structure to achieve the best results.

One of the most important aspects of job evaluation is that it focuses on job content--not the individual incumbents and their level of performance on the job. It also addresses the normal work environment, and not the unusual or emergency assistance that may infrequently occur on the job.

METHOD	ADVANTAGES	DISADVANTAGES
RANKING	°Least expensive °Little developmental time °Flexible	°Difficult to minimize bias °Lacks year-to-year continuity °Difficult to relate dissimilar job families °Lacks professional acceptance
PAIRED COMPARISON	°Quick and simple to develop and install °Mgmt. and employee participation enhances acceptance °Identifies bias or inconsistencies in evaluation	°Appears complicated °Assumes objectivity by evaluators °Requires statistical paired comparison automated programming
POINT FACTOR	°Easy to use °Evaluates differences in numerical terms °Facilitates grade development °Not easy to manipulate °Objectivity enhanced °Acceptance is high	°Time consuming °Requires clerical detail

1. Hospital Job Evaluation Plan

For the purposes of this manual, the point factor method has been chosen. The objective of the evaluation plan is to provide a common and reliable framework which can measure the content of each job.
This technique was selected because it is relatively simple to use, easily understood, and responsive to the need to compare a large number of dissimilar positions in a fair and equitable manner. In addition, the evaluation plan expresses differences in relative job value in numerical terms and provides for the common grading of all jobs: professional, administrative or service.

The basic characteristic of the plan is that it measures job content in terms of four primary compensable elements:

- Skill
- Responsibility
- Working Conditions
- Effort

These elements are then broken down into ten component parts (factors) that are applied to each job evaluation. These factors are:

<u>Skill</u>

1. Mental Development
2. Work Experience
3. Judgment

Responsibility

4. Errors and Losses
5. Resource Utilization
6. Systems and Data
7. Interpersonal Relationships

Working Conditions

8. Work Environment
9. Hazards

Effort

10. Personal Demands

Each of the above ten factors is defined by differentiating degrees, each with a numeric or point value. For example, Factor 1- Mental Development has five degrees, each with an assigned point value ranging from 15- 75 points.

The assigned point value ranges for the factors are:

Factors	Point Value Minimum	Point Value Maximum
Skill (40-200)		
1. Mental Development	15	75
2. Work Experience	15	75
3. Judgment	10	50
Responsibility (45-225)		
4. Errors and Losses	10	50
5. Resource Utilization	10	50
6. Systems and Data	10	50
7. Interpersonal Relationships	15	75

Factors	Point Value Minimum	Point Value Maximum
Working Conditions (10-50)		
8. Work Environment	5	25
9. Hazards	5	25
Effort (10-50)		
10. Personal Demands	10	50

Generally, the objectivity associated with this approach appeals to employees generating acceptance. The use of the ten factors suggests greater equity because it allows more functions of the hospital, such as service and administrative jobs, to be represented. Also, the ten factors and their weighting are stable, which gives credibility to this technique.

2. Job Evaluation Methodology

The following are the four basic job evaluation methods, which are divided into different classes:

1. Ranking method
2. Job classification method
3. Factor comparison method
4. Point method

The four methods can be divided into two groups of non-quantitative measures and quantitative evaluation measures.

Nonquantitative evaluation measures

The ranking and job classification methods are placed in this group. They briefly describe the job, including the duties, responsibilities, difficulties, and qualifications.

The Ranking Method

Ranking, the simplest method, also known as the "order of importance" system, is the oldest method used to determine the economic nature of a job. All jobs in the organization are ranked (compared or evaluated) on the basis of their overall importance to the organization. Grade levels are sometimes defined after the jobs have been ranked. This method is used in very small organizations. Generally, little or no attempt is made to break the job down with specific weighted rating factors. Ranking may be arranged by title only, or by combining title, job content, and compensating rates. The title of each job is placed on a card, which may contain job content, to facilitate judgment as to which job is more or less important in relation to other jobs.

The Job Classification Method

The job classification method is also known as the grading method. The idea behind this system is the belief that any number of jobs can be sorted out and classified into a number of predetermined classes, grades, or groups on the basis of some common denominators that run through the jobs. The common denominators are often levels of responsibilities, abilities, skills, knowledge, and duties. The job classes or grades are arranged (ranked) in an overall order of importance according to the common denominators.

The Factor Comparison Method

The factor comparison method is known as the "key job system." It has some characteristics of the ranking and the job classification system, but differs considerably in structure and application. The factor comparison method is more widely used than the ranking and the job classification method. Five evaluation factors are believed to exist in all jobs: skill, responsibility, physical effort, mental effort, and working conditions. All jobs should be compared to those critical factors. The basic idea of factor comparison is that all jobs should be compared and evaluated independently according to each of the evaluation factors. Thus, all jobs are compared independently five different times, once for each factor. For example, jobs are compared and ranked in the order they require skill--from the most to the least. All jobs are likewise compared and ranked according to the responsibility, physical effort, mental effort and working conditions of the job. The five separate rankings are then assigned monetary values. When the five values are added together, they result in each job having an overall monetary value or a base-rate price. The heart of this system of job evaluation is the use of "key jobs." "Key jobs" are those well-known jobs (such as registered nurse, medical technologist, nurse's aide) which over time have become standards of comparison because they do not change much. These jobs are first processed through the factor comparison system and then used as benchmarks for evaluating the remaining jobs.

<u>The Point Method</u> is used in the book and is the basis of the recommended job evaluation method.

3. Evaluation of Benchmark Jobs - Benchmark positions should be selected prior to the first job evaluation committee meeting. Benchmark positions are:

- Well known
- Highly populated
- Representative of different departments
- Representative of jobs from high to low in the current hierarchy of jobs
- Easily surveyed in the external job market

A good selection of benchmark jobs should encompass approximately 15% of the hospital's total number of job titles. Jobs commonly used as benchmarks include:

- Head Nurse
- RN
- LPN
- Nursing Assistant
- Unit Clerk
- Physical Therapist
- Medical Technologist
- Laboratory Section Supervisor
- Radiologic Technician
- Respiratory Therapist
- EKG or EEG Technician
- Department Secretary
- Dietitian
- Food Service Aide

- Housekeeping or Dietary Supervisor
- Housekeeper
- Medical Records Technician
- Medical Records Clerk
- File Clerk
- Admitting Clerk
- Credit and Collections Representative
- Medical Transcriber
- Telephone Operator
- Maintenance Supervisor
- Maintenance Mechanic
- Accounts Payable Clerk
- Payroll Clerk
- Business Office Supervisor

a. Preparation for job evaluation committee meeting-prior to the first job evaluation committee meeting, a delegated member of the committee must:

- Prepare a copy of the evaluation plan for each member of the committee.

- Schedule a quiet, private and comfortable room to meet where members may sit around a table.

- Assure that job documentation for the benchmark jobs is complete and that a copy is made for each member.

- Confirm that all members will be present and that they understand that all discussions are confidential and no interruptions, such as phone calls, will be permitted during the sessions.

- Provide a set of 3" x 5" cards with a job title printed on top of each card (one card for each benchmark job).

There is a considerable amount of recordkeeping and documentation involved in the evaluation process. If possible, a job evaluation committee recorder should be appointed, generally from the personnel department, who can be entrusted with a great deal of confidential information. Recordkeeping responsibilities will include:

- Preparation of materials for each session.
- Documentation of the basis for each evaluation.
- Maintaining a current list of each job's point value by:
  - total points (high to low)
  - by factor
  - by department

The maintenance of these various documents and the availability of this information to the committee at each session clearly increases the consistency and objectivity of the evaluation judgment for each factor.

In applying a job evaluation plan, a number of approaches may be taken. The job evaluation plan may be administered, for example, by:

- A personnel representative such as the personnel manager or job analyst.

- The institution administrator.

- A committee composed of institution management.

To achieve a maximum amount of acceptance and objective results, a committee approach is recommended. The evaluation committee should be made up of management personnel who are knowledgeable about the hospital's organizational structure and the interrelationships of the various departments. In addition, the committee should be representative of the major hospital functions. The size of the committee will vary but generally should be limited to six or seven members. A typical committee might consist of functional heads from:

- Nursing
- Technical Services
- Medical Records
- Plant Operations
- Food Services
- Personnel

b. Using the job documentation previously developed, the committee evaluates the benchmark jobs. The process generally proceeds as follows:

- A benchmark job description is selected and read aloud to the committee.

- Each committee member votes for a particular degree in Factor 1 either by written or oral vote.

- Votes are counted and discussion ensues regarding any differences in interpretation of the degree. It is through these discussions that perceptions of the job are shared and the interpretation of the degrees is defined further.

- Majority rules in the final determination of the appropriate degree, and it is documented.

- Each bencmark is read and evaluated on Factor 1.

- Index cards with benchmark job titles are arranged from high to low in order of assigned points for Factor 1, and tested for their appropriateness.

- The same process is followed for each factor for all benchmarks and is tested after each one to check for the consistent validity of each factor.

- Total point values are computed for each job. Job cards are arranged high to low, and reviewed for the appropriateness of the differences in relative job values. The higher the points, the higher the eventual pay grade.

- Adjustments to the total point value are made only if an individual factor change is justified and consistent with the other benchmarks for that particular factor.

It should be understood that this process is not scientific. It is, however, a systematic framework for making judgments. It should be noted that consistency and accuracy generally improves with use. Initially, the process proceeds slowly while the committee becomes familiar with the definitions of the degrees and begins to relate these definitions to their specific environment. Proficiency increases, however, and the evaluation process proceeds more quickly. Committee members should be cautioned at this point not to discuss the job evaluations outside the meetings due to the fact that the evaluations are subject to adjustment prior to final review.

Once the benchmark positions have been evaluated, they become the basis or reference points for all the remaining jobs and, in the future, any new or changed jobs. They are truly the foundation for all other evaluations.

4. <u>Evaluation of Non-Benchmark Jobs</u>

After the benchmarks have been set, each additional job is evaluated in total by referencing a benchmark job for each factor and documenting the job on the form titled "Basis for Evaluation."

The responsibility for evaluating the remaining jobs may rest with the committee, which will continue to meet on a scheduled basis, or may be assigned to the personnel representative. In the latter case, personnel would generally seek the help of the respective committee members when evaluating their functional area. These tentative evaluations would later be brought to the committee for review and approval.

After the evaluation of all jobs is complete and the committee is satisfied with the arrangement of jobs from highest to lowest, based upon their point value, a final list is presented to the administrator or CEO for review. It should be recognized, however, that any adjustments made at this point are generally minimal if the committee has been objective in its evaluation judgments.

5. <u>Evaluation of Generic Jobs</u>

To demonstrate the actual application of the Hospital Job Evaluation Plan included in this manual, the jobs which were previously discussed under Generic Hospital Job Descriptions have been evaluated and documented in Appendix A. These evaluations may be used in two ways:

- As a model or reference in the actual application of the plan.
- As established benchmarks that other jobs may be slotted against.

D. Job Grading

Grading is the grouping of jobs with substantially equal relative value, as determined through job evaluation, for the purpose of establishing fair pay levels. As mentioned earlier, the point evaluation method easily facilitates the establishment of pay grades. The higher the point value the higher the pay scale.

These job grades form the basis of the salary structure to which a salary range will be applied.

In setting the point range spreads that determine the individual job grades, a number of considerations are taken into account:

- The natural groupings or breaks in point values.

- The relationships between jobs in the same job family.

- The relationship between jobs with reporting relationships.

- The relationship between similar jobs which transcend departmental lines.

One basic rule is generally followed in setting the point ranges. This rule is that the point spread should either stay constant or increase as the grade level increases. For example, in the evaluations of the generic hospital descriptions, the total point values range from 155 to 475.

The following grades were established for these jobs and the point average and point spreads are shown:

Grade	Point Range	Point Spread
11	155 and below	-
12	160 - 180	20
13	185 - 205	20
14	210 - 230	20
15	235 - 255	20
16	260 - 280	20
17	285 - 310	25
18	315 - 340	25
19	345 - 370	25
20	375 - 405	30
21	410 - 440	30
22	445 - 475	30

In Grade 11, the lowest grade, the point spread was set at 155 and below to designate the first group of entry level jobs. The next group, or Grade 12, ranges from 160-180 or a 20 point spread. This group recognized the natural break in points between the Switchboard Operator at 175 and Nursing Assistant at 190 that will now fall into the next grade--Grade 13.

As can be seen, point spreads remain at 20 points until Grade 17 at which time it increases to 25. The next change occurs in Grade 20 when it increased to 30 and remains at this spread for the rest of the grades utilized in this example. At no time does the point spread decrease below the spread assigned to the previous grade.

After the initial setting of grades has been established, each grouping should be examined as a unit for compatibility. For example, if the Staff Nurse falls into the same grade as the Head Nurse, obviously the point spreads are not falling correctly or one of the positions was evaluated improperly.

As in job evaluations, the job grading is not a scientific process. But if the evaluation plan has been applied systematically and consistently, significant differences in point values should be easily determined and form the basis for establishing a fair set pay level.

POSITION SUMMARY QUESTIONNAIRE

EXHIBIT II-1A

POSITION TITLE: Respiratory Therapist (Certified) NAME: Jane Smith DATE: 3/12/81

NAME OF SUPERIOR/TITLE: Sue Brown, Director of Respiratory Technology DEPT.: Respiratory Therapy - First

PRIMARY PURPOSE OF FUNCTION OF YOUR POSITION - Write one or two sentences which summarize the purpose of your job

Perform various therapeutic treatments, including iron lungs, oxygen, catheters, canneuas and incubators

TYPICAL RESPONSIBILITIES OR DUTIES - List the most important duties. Include, if appropriate, responsibilities for equipment, product, safety, and work of others. Five to seven duties usually cover most jobs. Please use this form only - more space is provided on the next page.

ORDER OF IMPORTANCE (1,2,3, etc*)	WHAT IS DONE? (Begin with an Action Word**)	WHY IS IT DONE?	PERCENT OF TIME SPENT WEEKLY
1	Administer oxygen to patient	Facilitate breathing	20%
1	Administer therapeutic gases to patient	Comply with physician's orders	30%
1	Administer aerosol medications and treatments	For diagnostic and therapeutic reasons	5%
1	Perform chest physlotherapy, postural drainage, incentive spero-mety, and basic pulmonary functions	Comply with physician's orders	3%

*The number "1" being most important

**NOTE: Examples - Supervise, review, plan, analyze, type, calculate, lift, transport, tag, mark, check, etc.

TYPICAL RESPONSIBILITIES OR DUTIES - (Continued)

EXHIBIT II-1A

ORDER OF IMPORTANCE (1,2,3, etc*)	WHAT IS DONE? (Begin with an Action Word**)	WHY IS IT DONE?	PERCENT OF TIME SPENT WEEKLY
1	Drain and analyze arterial blood	Comply with physician's orders	3%
1	Enter treatments on patient charts, Chart patient information	Comply with physician's orders	10%
1	Observe patient for any adverse reactions during treatment	Comply with physician's orders	20%
3	Keep adequate supplies of gases, medications; keep equipment clean and sterilized	Comply with physician's orders	4%
2	Serve as team member of cardeopulmonary resuscitation team	Hospital Policy	4%

SKILL

QUALIFICATIONS, EXPERIENCE AND JUDGMENT - List here specific minimum requirements that one must possess to satisfactorily perform the duties of this position.

Educational and/or Professional Qualifications:	Certification as Registered Respiratory Therapist	Why? (Your opinion) Required by Joint Commission
Previous Job Experience	None	Why?
Other Special Training		Why?
Judgment (Decisions made independent of supervision)		Why?
Initiative/Ingenuity (Required to Fulfill Duties)		Why?

EXHIBIT II-1A

RESPONSIBILITY

CONTACTS WITH IMMEDIATE SUBORDINATES -

Nature of contacts with those under direct supervision of this position; such as assign work projects, review job performance, recommend wage increases, hire, take disciplinary action, etc.

IMMEDIATE SUBORDINATES

NUMBER	POSITION TITLE AND NAME*
None	

*One or two names only.

CONTACTS INSIDE AND OUTSIDE ORGANIZATION -

List those contacts other than contacts with subordinates. Describe the frequency (e.g. constantly, daily, occasionally). Also, state reason for contact; i.e., what is accomplished as a result of the contact.

IN-HOUSE AND OUTSIDE CONTACTS

DEPARTMENT, AGENCY, OFFICE, TITLE, ETC.	FREQUENCY	REASON FOR CONTACT
Patients	Daily	Administer treatment
Nursing Department	Daily	Coordinate activities

EXHIBIT II-1A

EQUIPMENT, MATERIALS, VALUABLES OR CONFIDENTIAL MATERIAL— List items you use or handle (respirator, welding materials, typewriter, paint, drugs, jewelry, money, medical records, credit reports).

ITEM	WHAT ARE YOUR DUTIES RELATED TO THE ITEM?
Therapeutic gas and mist inhalation equipment, i.e., masks, tents, catheters, canneuas and incubators, cylinders of gas, hand tools, etc.	Operates and monitors equipment, disassembles, cleans and sterilizes equipment

WORKING CONDITIONS AND EFFORT

WORK ENVIRONMENT AND SCHEDULE - List conditions which tend to be disagreeable, such as cold, heat, noise, fumes, dirt, water, weekend or irregular hours; describe the frequency (e.g., constantly, daily, occasionally).

CONDITION	WHERE DOES IT COME FROM? WHY ARE YOU EXPOSED TO IT?	FREQUENCY
Smells, etc.	Patient rooms	Daily
Unscheduled overtime as required	Heavy patient loads	As required
Evening, night and weekend shifts	24-hour coverage required	As required

EXHIBIT II-1A

WORKING CONDITIONS AND EFFORT (CONTINUED)

HAZARDS AND ABUSE - List factors which physically endanger you, such as machinery, electricity, falls, radiation, disease, etc. List items which may be emotionally upsetting, such as irrational patient behavior, abuse from the public, etc. Describe the frequency (e.g., constantly, daily, occasionally).

FACTOR	WHERE DOES IT COME FROM? WHY ARE YOU EXPOSED TO IT?	FREQUENCY
Infection	Frequently exposed to various respiratory infections	Daily

EXHIBIT II-1B

POSITION DESCRIPTION
WRITER'S GUIDE

FOR

COMMUNITY HOSPITAL

OUTLINE

Section

I. INTRODUCTION

AHA Community Hospital has decided to update its formal salary program. You are being asked to play a key role in this program by writing your own job description.

This Position Description Writer's Guide is designed to help each of you understand the assigned task, and develop the skill needed to accomplish it. To gain the most from this manual, you should read it thoroughly and complete the exercises as directed. The salary program is directed toward the following goals:

1. Internal Equity. To provide a salary range for each position that fairly and objectively reflects its value relative to other positions within the organization.
2. External Competitiveness. To provide a salary range for each position that will enable us to attract and retain the technical and managerial talent required to achieve organization goals.
3. Personal Motivation. To motivate each employee toward a specific achievement of individual position responsibilities through the application of salary administration guidelines which recognize different degrees of performance with differing salary rewards, thus stimulating and sustaining excellence in individual performance.
4. Continuity. To provide a program with the capability of responding to changes in organization, job design and external market influence through:
   a. Revision of job descriptions where job content has substantially changed;
   b. Preparation of descriptions for new jobs;
   c. Periodic reviews of positions;
   d. Annual review of salary administration against external comparisons.

The development of properly written job descriptions is the cornerstone of this program. So, to guarantee the high quality of workmanship that is necessary for success, we request each of you to put forth your best effort in writing your own position description.

II. DIRECTIONS

The material which follows is intended and designed to achieve several objectives.

1. To provide you with background material describing the format of the position description you will write to fulfill the requirements of the salary administration systems. Therefore, it is important that you:

   a. Read this Guide thoroughly.

   b. Understand the material contained in the Guide.

2. To provide written exercises which will enhance your understanding of the material and point to its practical application in the development of a formal written description. Again, it is important that you:

   a. Complete these exercises.

   b. Write them out completely and in detail as instructed, because the final position description will be used by the Hospital in establishing its salary program.

3. To provide you with a tool for your use in writing your own position description.

III. POSITION DESCRIPTION

It is critical that all position descriptions be written in a standard, concise and meaningful format.

Thus, this section of the Guide will deal with the format you will use in writing your description and the manner in which you should integrate the information into a well-organized position description.

1. General Format. Each position description will contain five sections.

   a. Heading - contains basic facts, such as job title, name, superior's title, etc.

   b. Position Purpose - a summary statement of what the position is designed to accomplish.

   c. Job Duties - a narrative description of the position's duties, challenges, departmental relationships, etc.

   d. Prime Responsibilities - a list of major end results the job is designed to accomplish.

   e. Skill and/or Qualifications - a statement of skill or knowledge required and educational or professional qualifications or experience desired.

All of this information will be written carefully and concisely in 2½ to 3 pages. Thus, a large part of the position description writer's task is to sift through the numerous activities, problems, interrelationships, and other important job information to determine what should be used and how it can be tightly woven together.

The remainder of this section of the Guide expands on the format of the five portions of the position description. Before going on, however, turn to the back of this Guide and review the last 3 pages. As you study through the remainder of this section, you will be asked to develop portions of you own description on these pages.

2. Heading. The top of the first page shows the way the heading should appear. Each of the blanks should be filled in as follows:

   Position - official title of the position.

   Incumbent - name of the person holding the position (your name).

   Department - function or unit in which the position is found.

   Reports to - title of your superior.

   Date - month and year of the position description.

   Written by - position description writer (your name).

   Approved by - (1) your signature
   (2) your immediate supervisor's signature (after you have finished writing description).

   EXERCISE: Fill in as much of the heading information as you can.

3. Position Purpose. This section requires a brief, undetailed, specific statement of why the position exists. In other words, what is its primary purpose of being included in the organization?

   The reason for such a succinct statement at the very outset is so the reader can immediately understand the position's overall role in the organization.

You may get this information by asking yourself a question like "What is the basic purpose of this position?," or "What part of the Department's total objectives do I accomplish in my position?"

On the other hand, if you aren't used to thinking in those terms, you may have to think about your job in detail first, and then arrive at such a statement. Usually, you will have a pretty good idea of the Position Purpose and it will simply be a matter of finding the correct phraseology and words. Typically, the statement is similar to the one you make or say to a neighbor or relative when they ask, "What do you do at AHA Community?"

This section will not exceed three or four lines. It is limited to one sentence or two at the most.

The Position Purpose of head of a personnel function might be as follows:

> "Acquire, develop and maintain the quality and quantity of employees needed through the development, recommendation and implementation of sound personnel policies and practices."

Notice that the Position Purpose does not include a detailed list of "how" the activity is accomplished, nor a lengthy review of the operation, its problems, nor the personal opinions of the person in the position (all of which you may first think about as an answer to this direct question about Position Purpose).

An illustration of how not to write a Position Purpose of the personnel function would be:

> "Acquire, develop and retain the number of good people needed to operate the hospital by using a variety of recruiting sources (but not an agency where you have to pay a fee); by demonstrating to the employees that you are interested in them by providing benefits such as a Christmas party for their children, as well as the regular review of benefits, etc."

You will have to distill what is relevant, use it judiciously and in meaningful language.

EXERCISE: Write the position purpose for your job. You should be able to write this (and each subsequent section of your position description) fairly quickly.

4. Job Duties. This section provides a clear, concise overview of the position. It incorporates the bulk of information you will gather. The length of the section varies depending on the complexity of the position, but usually covers about two pages total (some of page 1, all of page 2, and a portion of page 3). Even that amount of space, however, requires tight concise writing.

   The organization of this section generally follows the topical order listed below:

   a. Functions performed by you personally.

   b. Composition of supporting staff and their position purpose (one sentence).

   c. Major challenges to the position.

   d. Controls on the position's freedom to perform and solve problems related to the job.

   e. Necessary contacts (inside and outside) of the hospital.

   f. Measurements of effectiveness of the position.

   The following list of items to cover will be particularly helpful in writing the Job Duties of your position:

   a. Functions performed by you personally

      - Functions you perform yourself (as distinguished from those performed through subordinates or in concert with others).

b. <u>Organization of subordinate activities</u>

- A summary of each subordinate position purpose or function;
- Number of employees supervised.

c. <u>Major challenges to the position</u>

- Nature and variety of most typical problems;
- The greatest challenges in the job.

d. <u>Controls on your freedom to act and solve job problems</u>

- Types of problems that must be referred to a superior for resolution or for approval for the incumbent's recommended solution;
- Authority the position has for:

  hiring and firing
  making capital expenditures
  purchasing supplies and services
  changing salaries

- Principal rules, regulations, precedents and controls within which the position operates.

e. <u>Contacts inside and outside the organization</u>

- Your most significant contacts with other areas within the organization - frequency and purpose;
- Your most significant contacts outside the organization - frequency and purpose;
- Types of problems you must consult with others to resolve.

f. Performance Measurement

- What are the end results which will serve as the base for evaluating the performance of you and your unit?

EXERCISE: Write the Job Duties section for your position. Start each one in a new paragraph. The list of action verbs may be helpful to you. (p. 74.)

5. Prime Responsibilities

These are statements of the "end results" of the position. The term "end results" does not mean a list of activities or duties, but rather fairly broad statements of what the job is structured to acomplish. Therefore, they are end results oriented rather than activity oriented. Consider this sample illustration for a homemaker.

Job Duties	Prime Responsibilities
- Wax furniture - Make beds - Sweep floors - Empty garbage	Ensure that the house is maintained in a clean and orderly fashion by executing household duties.

You can see that specific job duties fall into general groups which describe "end results." The responsibility is written with the "end result" first, i.e., ensure that the house...

As the example illustrates, a prime responsibility implies Action. Each statement should relate to an "end result" that must be accomplished. In the above example, the end result or response was "providing a clean home."

Each job is answerable for certain actions and the consequence of those actions--these are the job's responsibilities. For each position, there are certain "end results" which are accomplished by subordinate positions, but there are also certain "end results" which can only be accomplished by you in the job being described.

The responsibilities of a subordinate position may be included within a single aspect of a superior position. In fact, it may be that a certain element, which is only considered as a general responsibility for a superior, constitutes a number of specific responsibilities for a subordinate. For instance, in many cases a department head must have certain records to accomplish particular "end results." In that position, record keeping may not be an "end result" at all, but there is frequently a subordinate job, the major purpose of which is timely and accurate maintenance of records.

The responsibilities listed in a position description state specific major "end results" expected for the position; i.e., the responsibilities are required to accomplish the basic function of the job. Clearly stated and understood responsibilities are necessary in order for employees to work effectively toward the accomplishment of desired Hospital, department or unit goals. For example, the statement "assists field operations" refers to an activity and lacks meaning in terms of what the position is expected to achieve through assistance. Similarly, "maximize utilization and minimize cost" is not a meaningful responsibility because it is vague and too general.

Responsibilities should be worded so that they will almost automatically lead to thoughts of MEASUREMENT. That is, they do not contain measures themselves but should provide clues to where measures might be found. For example, "maximum utilization" might be reworded, "achieve work force utilization objective." The latter leads to measures against an established objective whereas the former does not.

For Department Head positions, the focus of responsibilities is on the elements of management-- organizing, staffing, motivating, planning, policy making, coordinating, controlling-- and should reflect the basic areas of "end results," such as utilization, work force development, costs, etc., which are essential for the hospital's survival and growth.

Beyond the specific responsibilities for a job, experience has shown that the incumbent in any position should be responsible for achieving specified "end results" without adverse effects on the performance of others. This is necessary since you may achieve desired results, but in a way that is only in your own or your department's self-interests rather than the broad interests of the Hospital.

There are a select number of key areas which relate to the accomplishment of total Hospital objectives. They are not statements of how to do something. You should note that each statement must include: an end result which is to be accomplished, action verb(s) that describes the type of action taken, and a function upon which the action is taken. These three elements--end result, action verb and function--are essential to a good statement of responsibility. Where applicable, the responsibility will also include the constraint put on the performance of a given responsibility.

An example of a responsibility for a Personnel Director which includes all four elements:

END RESULT	Meet hospital's work force requirements.
ACTION VERB(S)	Planning and assuring.
FUNCTION	Timely recruitment of competent exempt, non-exempt and hourly personnel.
CONSTRAINT	With due consideration to the special specifications of Department Heads.

In summary, a responsibility should be:

A basic "end result" expected from the position under consideration.

Clearly worded to emphasize action.

Stated in such a way that allows performance to be measured objectively, in quantifiable terms whenever possible.

Responsibilities should not be:

- Statements of day-to-day details, duties, or responsibilities;
- So broad and vague their meaning is unclear;
- A combination of several major end results.

For most positions write down 5 to 8 responsibilities.

EXERCISE: Write the most important responsibilities of your postion. If you need some help getting started, make a detailed list of your position's responsibilities and then try to group them together under Prime Responsibilities.

Analyze each statement in terms of the following criteria:

- Does the statement include all necessary elements - end result, action verb, function and where applicable, a constraint?
- Is the "end result" described by the statement timeless, that is, applicable no matter who holds the position, or when the position is held?
- Does the action verb (provide, review, administer, assure) correctly reflect the position's role and authority?
- Does the statement give any indication where to look for measures?
- Is the statement sufficiently specific to measure performance against?

If you have answered NO to any of the above questions for any one of your statements, rewrite it.

6. Skill and/or Qualifications. In this section, identify bona fide requirements of skill or knowledge, as well as specific educational or professional qualifications or equivalent experience desired. This would include, for example, licensure requirements, state accreditation, professional organizations, degrees required, or experience. Avoid stating as requirements those skills or qualifications that are merely desired and not necessary to perform the position's functions.

IV. SUMMARY

All there is to a vitally important task of position description writing is summed up in:

- Creativity and probingly thinking about the pertinent areas of your position.
- Understanding the information that is important and recording it without editorializing, evaluating, etc.
- Taking a clear, organized view of your job which can be integrated into a properly written position description.

Thank you for taking time to complete this assignment.

V. ACTION WORDS

Accumulate
Administer
Advise
Analyze
Appraise
Approve
Ascertain
Assign
Assure
Audit
Authorize

Budget

Calculate
Check
Collaborate
Collect
Compile
Complete
Conduct
Consolidate
Consult
Contact
Contribute
Control
Coordinate
Counsel

Delegate
Design
Determine
Develop
Dictate
Direct
Discuss
Distribute

Ensure
Establish
Evaluate
Examine
Execute
Expedite

Facilitate
Follow-up
Forecast
Formulate
Function
Furnish

Gather
Give

Implement
Improve
Inform
Initiate
Inspect
Issue
Interpret
Interview
Inventory
Investigate

Maintain
Make
Manage
Motivate

Notify

Obtain
Operate

Participate
Plan
Present
Produce
Provide

Receive
Recommend
Record
Reject
Release
Report
Represent
Review
Revise

Schedule
Secure
See
Serve
Service
Sign
Specify
Standardize
Store
Structure
Study
Submit
Supply
Supervise
Survey

Take
Train

Verify

POSITION DESCRIPTION

Date:____________________ Position:________________________

Written by:____________________ Incumbent:________________________

Approved by: (1)_____________ Department:________________________

(2)_____________ Reports to:________________________

Position Purpose:

Job Duties:

POSITION DESCRIPTIONS

Job Duties (Continued)

Prime Responsibilities

Skill and/or Qualifications

SECTION III

MARKET COMPETITIVENESS

A. The Purpose and Use of Wage and Salary Surveys

- Wage and salary surveys are used by hospital personnel representatives and administration:

  1. To determine the "market value" of hospital jobs.

  2. To determine the competitiveness of current hospital pay levels.

  3. To generate data from which an existing compensation structure may be adjusted or revised for competitiveness.

  4. To establish a basis to compare in-house relativities with those of other organizations.

- There are basically two types of wage and salary surveys:

  1. General surveys of pay levels for all areas of the hospital (usually done annually).

  2. Specialty surveys to obtain information on a particular professional field or area of the hospital (done on an "as needed" basis).

B. Available (Published) Wage and Salary Surveys

There are many wage and salary surveys for hospital positions conducted on an annual basis by various organizations, public and private. Some advantages of using published surveys are that they are:

- Readily available at little or no cost.

- Periodic and repetitive.

- Available for most types of positions.

- Include a large number of participants.

- Provide a good indication of general compensation trends.

- Do not require much time to utilize.

Some disadvantages of using published surveys are that:

- Information is frequently out-of-date by the time of publication, and/or undated.

- Positions surveyed may or may not compare with positions at the hospital, and frequently insufficient information is given for job matching.

- Participant number and mix varies greatly.

- Quality of job comparisons and validity of results is unknown.

Due to the advantages listed, published surveys are a useful tool to determine general compensation trends. For a partial list of available surveys, see Exhibit III-1. When using external surveys, it is important to note <u>when</u> the survey data was collected. If it is more than one or two months old, the survey data should be adjusted up by the approximate percentage market movement in the time elapsed. For the last few years, hospital salaries have been moving approximately 8-10 percent per year. To interpret information received through these surveys, see Section D of this Section, "How to Analyze Survey Results".

C. How to Design and Run a Self-Conducted Salary Survey

By far the best wage and salary data is gained from self-conducted surveys. By designing and conducting their own surveys, hospital management can control who is surveyed, what is surveyed, and how carefully data is collected. As a result, these surveys can be used with a high degree of confidence.*

1. How to Determine Survey Participants--Defining the Job Market - The first step in designing a salary survey is to decide what other institutions should be invited to participate. Frequently, hospital administration and/or the governing body has definite ideas about whom they wish, and do not wish, to compete with in the job market. For example, some organizations do not wish to compete with union pay levels, but others feel it is necessary. The market definition should be discussed and determined with hospital senior management.

   The answers to the following questions will help in determining the job market, and what survey participants to include.

   Q. What is the comparative policy of the hospital--is it the wage leader or wage follower?

   A. If the hospital wishes to be a wage leader, it is important to survey the highest paying institutions in the area. If the competitive strategy is middle-of-the-road, it is important to chose participants representing all pay levels in the market.

*However, such surveys may increase the hospital's exposure to antitrust liability. See Section E of this chapter.

Q. Who does the hospital directly compete with to recruit personnel?

A. Obviously, other local hospitals should be surveyed. For certain positions, such as maintenance jobs, it may be necessary to survey organizations outside the hospital industry. For others, particularly higher level positions, the job market region becomes geographically larger, and more institutions should be included.

Q. Number of participants?

A. As a rule, at least five participants should be included to develop meaningful, worthwhile results. When the number is less than this, it is frequently helpful to supplement the data with published survey results. Obviously, when more participants are included in the survey, the data base is larger and survey results are more representative of overall job market conditions.

Q. Promise of feedback?

A. Frequently, the only way a survey designer can enlist the participation of other institutions is to promise a final report of survey results, as well as to maintain confidentiality of participant data. When contacting prospective participants, the fulfillment of these promises should be guaranteed.

Q. Sample constancy?

A. If the hospital wishes to use self-conducted surveys on a regular basis, the participants selected should be relatively consistent so that survey results may be meaningfully compared from one year to the next.

2. <u>What to Ask in a Salary Survey</u> - In conducting a survey, the survey designer has total freedom in selecting what general information and positions to include in the survey. Sometimes, surveys are conducted to research a particular position or problem, but most frequently, general surveys are conducted on an annual basis to assist in determining adjustments in salary/wage ranges to remain competitive in the coming year.

In a general survey, there are usually two sections:

The general questionnaire

Job data

<u>The General Questionnaire</u> - General questions frequently asked of survey participants are the following:

- Number of beds?

- Number of employees?

- Basic type of salary program - merit, longevity or both? (How does it work?)

- Are there any special structures or compensation policies for a particular group of employees?

- What positions are represented by a union?

- When were salary ranges last adjusted, and how much did they move?

- When will salary ranges next be adjusted, and how much is it anticipated they will move?

- What is the hospital's shift differential policy?

- What are related employee benefits?

- What are associated policies and procedures?

- Are there other forms of direct pay, such as incentives or bonuses?

- What are the turnover statistics?

- What are the characteristics of the compensation structure?

Hospital management may also use this time to ask information about benefits or other issues that are currently surfacing as employee concerns in the institution. For example, employees may be asking questions about adding dental coverage to existing benefit plans, and the survey can be used as an opportunity to find out what other institutions are doing in this area. See sample survey questionnaire in Exhibit III-2.

Job Data - The bulk of a salary/wage survey requests specific pay information for specific positions.

a. What Positions to Survey -

- Choose Benchmarks--In a general survey, it is best to select benchmark positions, representing as many pay levels and departments of the hospital as possible. See Section II for a complete definition of how to identify benchmark positions.

- Choose Jobs Easy to Match Outside--Be sure to select jobs that are likely to be easily matched at the participant organizations. If a job has developed unique responsibilities, not normally associated with that title or field, it will likely be very difficult to find a good job match elsewhere in order to compare salary data.

- Choose Jobs that are Problems to Fill or Retain Employees--Several medical fields are currently undergoing unusual market situations. This may be because the field is new and relatively unstandardized. (A good example is Laboratory Technology with two- and four-year degree offerings.) Also, in many professions, job responsibilities are changing, such as in Nursing and Respiratory Therapy. In addition, many areas of the hospital suffer from a shortage of qualified personnel in the job market, and competitive salary ranges are especially important. Sometimes, it may be warranted to conduct a special survey for particular problem areas, such as salaries for a particular profession, to aid in developing ranges to attract and retain qualified personnel in these areas. Generally, these special surveys are conducted to acquire specific information in a particular area, and are not done on a regular basis.

b. <u>What Information to Ask</u> - Once the positions to be surveyed have been selected, the following information should be asked about each one:

- Salary range (minimum, midpoint and maximum; or timing and amount of steps if participant is on a lock-step program. See next section).

- Average paid salary?

- Actual high and low salaries?

- Number of incumbents in position

- How participant's position differs from survey description

It is important to include a brief job description on the survey form, whether the survey is being conducted over the phone, in person, or in written form to assure consistent job definition and good job matching. See Exhibit III-3 for a sample job survey form.

c. <u>How to Make a Job Match</u> - A survey is only as good as the closeness of the job comparison (job match). The biggest mistake in job matching is making the match strictly on the basis of job title. This frequently leads to comparing unlike jobs as institutions develop titling systems over the years which are unique to their organization. For this reason, a brief description should always accompany the job being surveyed. Jobs should be matched on the basis of duties performed. If the basic job duties are the same, it will be a good salary comparison, regardless of the difference in job titles.

d. <u>Collection of Survey Information</u> - Survey data can be collected in three basic ways:

- Face-to-Face Interviews.
- Written Surveys.
- Telephone Surveys.

1. Face-to-Face Interviews - These are not generally used for large, general surveys, because of the time necessary to conduct them, but they are an excellent way to gain general data about the participant and information on "hard to match" jobs.

Advantages:

-- Assures the acquisition of a good understanding of the participant's compensation practices.

-- Allows for a thorough understanding of jobs and the quality of the job matches.

-- Survey results can be gathered relatively quickly.

Disadvantages:

-- On-site, face-to-face interviews are very time consuming for the survey interviewer.

-- Participants may not be willing to schedule a block of time.

2. Written Surveys are frequently used for the annual, general survey.

Advantages:

-- Written job descriptions are included for participant reference in job matching.

-- Written surveys are not as time consuming as personal interviews.

-- Participants may complete survey at their leisure (and be more willing to participate).

-- A great deal of information may be requested.

Disadvantages:

-- Frequently information is not returned from participants for three weeks or a month.

-- Participant matches must be relied upon.

-- Survey forms are frequently returned only partially completed.

3. Telephone Surveys are best for brief surveys requesting specific information.

Advantages:

-- Data can be gathered quickly.

Disadvantages:

-- Job matches are made hastily, and frequently with insufficient information.

-- Participants may have to gather data from sources not readily available.

e. Confidentiality/Survey Reporting

- Confidentiality - Many institutions will not participate in wage and salary surveys unless confidentiality is guaranteed. Confidentiality of participant wage and salary information must be respected. Therefore, individual participant data must be assigned a confidential code. The final report may contain a list of the participants, but does not reveal responses of individual institutions.

- Survey Report - In order to enlist the participant's cooperation, it is generally necessary to compile a final report of survey results for the participants. Generally, the data on each job should be averaged, highs and lows reported as well as number of matched incumbents recorded. See Exhibit III-4 for a sample survey final report.

D. How to Analyze Survey Results.

There are many statistical methods to analyze self-conducted and published survey results, but two of the most simple and meaningful are the following:

1. Bar Graphs - Plot bar graphs, by position, of salary ranges and average paid salaries. See Exhibit III-5 for sample bar graphs. This provides a good visual representation of current market position, particularly when presenting survey results to others who are not familiar with compensation terminology. It is also easy to determine if other participants use wider or smaller salary ranges, and if their average pay and starting salaries are comparable.

2. Average Paid Salary - Determine the average paid salary for each position, for all participants' data. This is a very useful number to determine current market position of hospital wages. Organizing the information according to internal grade structure helps identify whether there are problems with a particular job, a particular group of ranges, or the entire salary structure. See Exhibit III-6 for an example of this analysis.

   Please note that in some positions where there are very few incumbents, the longevity of the individuals may have great impact on the average paid salary. Such considerations should be taken into account when analyzing data.

Analyze starting wages to assure that in-house starting wage levels are competitive. Use responses to the general questionnaire to estimate market movement for the coming year, and market competitiveness of other compensation areas besides base pay.

Survey results and determination of current external job market conditions, combine with internal evaluation and relativity results, will determine a sound, internally equitable and externally competitive salary structure for the hospital. To see how this data is used in the development of a salary structure, see Section IV.

E. Antitrust Considerations

Antitrust laws at both the state and federal level prohibit concerted actions in restraint of trade. One of the traditional categories constituting "restraint of trade" is price-fixing. Concerted actions among competitors regarding costs, as components of prices, may be construed as a restraint of trade in the same manner as actual price-fixing. Thus, the issue arises as to whether the exchange of information among hospitals regarding salaries might subject such hospitals to antitrust liability.

In general, the exchange of business information, including salaries or even prices, is not in and of itself a violation of the antitrust laws. However, if the exchange can be shown to be the basis for an agreement or concerted action to affect prices or competition, it may be found to be an antitrust violation. Price standardization or stabilization constitutes an affect on prices for antitrust purposes.

In conducting salary surveys, then, a hospital should not use the results in any way that is suggestive of an attempt to fix costs (prices) or restrain trade. The key element in the antitrust analysis is the use of the results. Even a published government wage and salary survey could be the basis for an antitrust violation if competitors used it to reach an anti-competitive agreement. On the other hand, a hospital may gather salary information for its own management purposes without violating the antitrust laws, so long as such information is not used in any way as part of an agreement to restrain trade.

In addition to avoiding the use of salary survey results as a basis for discussions among competitors or other concerted actions which could trigger antitrust liability, hospitals seeking salary information should be aware of the following:

(1) The use of published surveys generally decreases antitrust risks, as it is more difficult to infer an agreement to restrain trade on the part of the users of such surveys.

(2) Surveys conducted or contracted for by particular hospitals should focus only on past or current salaries, not

plans for future salaries, as the latter more readily leads to an inference of concerted actions.

(3) Surveys drawing from a broad range of hospitals, rather than only direct competitors, also are less suggestive of anticompetitive behavior.

(4) Information gathered should be released only internally if at all possible. Obviously, it would be difficult to prove the existence of an agreement where only one party possesses the necessary information. If results must be disseminated in order to assure adequate participation in the survey, only aggregate statistics should be released, with the responses of individual hospitals kept confidential.

PUBLISHED SURVEYS FOR THE HEALTH CARE INDUSTRY

-- VARIOUS GOVERNMENT WAGE AND SALARY SURVEYS

- AREA WAGE SURVEY

- NATIONAL SURVEY OF PROFESSIONAL, ADMINISTRATIVE, TECHNICAL AND CLERICAL PAY
  Both available: Bureau of Labor Statistics, Department of Labor, 441 G street, N.W., Washington, D.C., 20212

-- GENERAL MANAGEMENT ASSOCIATION SURVEYS

- AMERICAN MANAGEMENT ASSOCIATION, "HOSPITAL AND HEALTH CARE REPORT"
  Available: Executive Compensation Service, American Management Association, 135 West 50 Street, New York, New York, 10020
- AMERICAN SOCIETY OF PERSONNEL ADMINISTRATORS
  Available: American Society of Personnel Administrators, 19 Church Street, Berea, Ohio, 44017

-- PRIVATE ORGANIZATION SURVEYS

- MANAGEMENT RESOURCES ASSOCIATION, INC.
  Available: Management Resources Association, Inc., 2421 North Mayfair Road, Milwaukee, Wisconsin, 53226
- BLUE CROSS-BLUE SHIELD NATIONAL SALARY SURVEY
  Available: Blue Cross-Blue Shield of Indiana, 120 West Market Street, Indianapolis, Indiana, 46204
- HOSPITAL COMPENSATION SERVICE
  Available: John R. Zabka Associates, 115 Watchung Drive, Hawthorne, New Jersey, 07506

-- STATE HOSPITAL ASSOCIATIONS AND AREA HOSPITAL COUNCILS

FOR THE MOST COMPLETE LIST OF AVAILABLE SURVEYS PUBLISHED, SEE <u>AVAILABLE PAY SURVEY REPORTS: AN ANNOTATED BIBLIOGRAPHY</u>, ABBOT, LARGER AND ASSOCIATES, P.O. BOX 275, PARK FOREST, ILLINOIS, 60466

AHA COMMUNITY HOSPITAL
WAGE & SALARY SURVEY GENERAL QUESTIONNAIRE

PARTICIPANT: ______________________________

1. Are any of the employees at your hospital represented by a union? ________ If so, which employee group(s)?
   ____
   Union: ______________________________

2. Do you have a merit program? ________ Who is eligible?
   ____
   Briefly, how does it work? ______________________________
   ____
   ____
   ____

3. When was your salary structure last reviewed? ________
   How much was adjusted? ________ %

4. When do you next plan to adjust your salary structure?
   ____
   How much do you anticipate they will move? ________ %

5. What is your shift differential policy? ________
   ____
   ____

6. Do you have length of service awards? ________ What are they? ______________________________
   ____
   ____

EXHIBIT III-3

JOB SURVEY REPORT

JOB TITLE: Respiratory Therapist

PARTICIPANT: ____________________

DEFINITION: Sets up and operates various types of oxygen and other therapeutic gas and inhalation equipment such as iron lungs, tents, masks, catheters, cannulas, and incubators, to administer prescribed doses of medicinal gases and aerosolized drugs. Prepares and maintains a chart for each patient. Cleans, inspects and tests inhalation therapy equipment.

HOW DOES YOUR JOB DIFFER?

CERTIFICATION REQUIRED: RRT Certification

NO.OF INCUMBENTS ____________

AVERAGE PAID SALARY ____________

ACTUAL PAID HIGH WAGE ____________

HIRING RATE ____________

ACTUAL PAID LOW WAGE ____________

SALARY RANGE:

____________ MIN

____________ MID

____________ MAX

COMMENTS:

EXHIBIT III-4

AHA COMMUNITY HOSPITAL

WAGE AND SALARY SURVEY

MARCH, 19XX

EXHIBIT III - 4

SAMPLE COVER LETTER FOR RETURNING SURVEY RESULTS

Dear ____________:

Enclosed are the results of the AHA Community Hospital Wage and Salary Survey for the Midville area. As you know, data was collected in March, and is expressed in hourly rates. Data was gathered from six area hospitals and the American Management Association Hospital and Health Care Report for our region, totalling 3,671 incumbents in the data base.

Survey participant data has been coded to retain confidentiality. Your survey code is __________.

Thank you so much for participating in our survey. We hope that the information will be as useful to you as it is to us. If you have any questions regarding the survey, please don't hesitate to give me a call at _____-__________.

Sincerely,

Personnel Director
AHA Community Hospital

EXHIBIT III-4

SUMMARY OF GENERAL QUESTIONNAIRE

PARTICIPANTS #	1	2	3	4	5	6
1. Any employees represented by Union?	YES LPN Techni-cal Unit	NO	NO	NO	NO	NO
2. Do you have a merit pro-ram?	NO	YES 6 month 12 month then annual 2.75% 1 stp 5.3% 2 stp (top 10%)	YES Merit and General	YES-up to Maximum of 6%	Special bonus for outstand-ing per-formance after 2 years of employment	YES-2-4% variation in annual increase based on merit
3. Last time salary ranges reviewed	JULY	JANUARY	JULY	JANUARY	JULY	JULY
% increase	10%	5%	9%	6-7%	9%	?
4. Next time salary ranges reviewed	JULY	JULY	JULY	JULY	JULY	JULY
% increase	?	3-5%	8%	? Cola	?	10%
5. Bonus or incentive plans	NONE	NONE	NONE	NONE	NONE	NONE
6. Shift differen-tial policy	% of base pay 30-60¢ 40-70¢	.41¢ RN .25¢ LPN .21¢ Tech .13¢ others	1% of Base Rate	6% 3-11 & 11-7 RNs 6% 38¢ 11-7 LPNs 6% 30¢ 11-7	Min. .20/ hour Max. .50/ hour	8% of current base salary
7. Do you have awards for length of service?	Ser-vice pins 5-10 15-20 25-30 Annual Dinner Hosp. week	Ser-vice pins 3-5-10 years dinner & 1 guest	Yes	Dinner 5-10-15 20-25 year	Yes	None

AHA Comm. Hosp. Wage /Salary Survey 3/15/xx

SURVEY : 2

POSITION	RESPONDENT DATA ACTUAL SALARIES LOW	AVERAGE	HIGH	NO. OF INCUMBTS	ALL PARTICANTS MINUS RESPONDENT ACTUAL SALARIES LOW	AVERAGE	HIGH	NUMBER OF INCMBT/PRTCPNT	
SECURITY OFFICER	5.36	6.60	7.72	10	4.40	6.16	7.32	74	6
SOCIAL SERVICE SEC	5.66	6.97	8.30	9	5.06	6.71	8.80	47	6
MED TRANSCRIBER	5.36	6.87	7.72	6	4.96	6.74	8.56	30	8
ACCTS PAYABLE CLERK	5.36	6.78	7.72	1	4.77	6.35	8.06	16	9
ADMITTING CLERK	5.36	6.30	7.72	11	4.63	5.92	7.87	71	9
CREDIT REPRESENTATIV	5.36	6.59	7.72	2	4.87	6.52	8.06	16	7
TELEPHONE OPERATOR	5.14	6.22	6.68	3	4.56	5.99	7.64	103	9
EKG TECHNICIAN	5.71	7.46	7.91	5	4.76	6.17	9.26	47	9
LAB TECHNOLOGIST	6.86	8.26	9.92	28	6.50	8.10	10.64	115	8
RESPIRATORY THERAPY	6.86	7.65	9.92	22	6.30	7.67	10.64	40	8
X RAY TECHNICIAN	6.87	8.78	9.92	8	6.40	7.97	10.64	91	9
SPECIAL PROC TECH					6.13	7.61	9.73	6	3
NUCLEAR MED TECH	6.86	8.43	9.92	5	5.77	7.91	13.75	15	8
PHYSICAL THERAPIST	6.83	8.26	10.30	4	6.50	8.13	17.01	43	9
OT TECHNICIAN	5.72	7.35	7.92	5	4.63	6.44	8.27	29	9
PHARMACIST	6.83	10.30	11.30	5	7.72	10.07	15.05	38	9
LPN	5.71	7.07	8.41	69	5.38	6.62	9.41	591	9
RN	7.33	8.67	10.81	259	6.66	8.31	12.26	1074	8
ASST HEAD NURSE	8.83	9.97	10.85	7	7.38	9.00	12.51	59	6
HEAD NURSE	9.30	11.30	13.81	12	7.61	9.82	12.85	92	7
LAB SECTION SUPV	10.72	10.72	10.72	5	6.20	10.40	14.03	20	6
BILLING SUPERVISOR	8.80	8.80	8.80	2	6.20	8.09	9.81	8	5
PAYABLE SUPERVISOR					5.13	8.06	9.59	5	5
				478				2630	9

EXHIBIT III-4

EXHIBIT III-4

AHA Comm. Hosp. Wage /Salary Survey 3/15/xx

COMPOSITE - ALL PARTICIPANTS

POSITION	ACTUAL SALARIES LOW	AVERAGE	HIGH	NUMBER OF INCMBT	/PRTCPNT
SECURITY OFFICER	4.40	6.22	7.72	84	7
SOCIAL SERVICE SEC	5.06	6.76	8.80	56	7
MED TRANSCRIBER	4.96	6.76	8.56	36	9
ACCTS PAYABLE CLERK	4.77	6.37	8.06	17	10
ADMITTING CLERK	4.63	5.97	7.87	82	10
CREDIT REPRESENTATIV	4.87	6.53	8.06	18	8
TELEPHONE OPERATOR	4.56	5.99	7.64	106	10
EKG TECHNICIAN	4.76	6.29	9.28	52	10
LAB TECHNOLOGIST	6.50	8.13	10.64	143	9
RESPIRATORY THERAPY	6.30	7.66	10.64	62	9
X RAY TECHNICIAN	5.40	8.04	10.64	99	10
SPECIAL PROC TECH	6.13	7.61	9.73	6	3
NUCLEAR MED TECH	5.77	8.04	13.75	20	9
PHYSICAL THERAPIST	6.50	8.14	17.01	47	10
OR TECHNICIAN	4.63	6.57	8.27	34	10
PHARMACIST	6.83	10.10	15.05	43	10
LPN	5.38	6.66	9.41	660	10
RN	6.66	8.38	12.26	1333	9
ASST HEAD NURSE	7.38	9.10	12.51	66	7
HEAD NURSE	7.61	9.99	13.81	104	8
LAB SECTION SUPV	6.20	10.46	14.03	25	7
BILLING SUPERVISOR	6.20	8.24	9.81	10	6
PAYABLE SUPERVISOR	5.13	8.06	9.59	5	5
				3108	10

EXHIBIT III-5

AHA Comm. Hosp. Wage /Salary Survey 3/15/xx

```
JOB: 44  ADMITTING CLERK          ESTABLISHED SALARY RANGES AND ACTUAL SALARIES - BY POSITION, AND BY PARTICIPANT

                              3.00      4.50      6.00      7.50      9.00     10.50     12.00     13.50     15.00     16.50     18.00
PARTICIPANTS  (INCUMBENTS)    +---------+---------+---------+---------+---------+---------+---------+---------+---------+---------+

     1           (  4)                      L.........A.H

     2           ( 11)                        L......A........H

     3           (  0)

     4           (  8)                     L.......A...........H

     5           ( 10)                        L..A.........H

     6           (  0)

     7           ( 12)                          L.A....H

     8           ( 10)                    L..........A.H

     9           (  6)                   L..A.............H

    10           (  8)                          L....A....H

    11           (  6)                       L..A......H

    12           (  7)                         L..A......H

                              +---------+---------+---------+---------+---------+---------+---------+---------+---------+---------+
                              3.00      4.50      6.00      7.50      9.00     10.50     12.00     13.50     15.00     16.50     18.00
```

EXHIBIT III-5

AHA Comm. Hosp. Wage /Salary Survey 3/15/xx

```
JOB: 119 EXECUTIVE HOUSEKEEPER        ESTABLISHED SALARY RANGES AND ACTUAL SALARIES - BY POSITION, AND BY PARTICIPANT

                              12400     17150     21900     26650     31400     36150     40900     45650     50400     55150     59900
PARTICIPANTS  (INCUMBENTS)    +---------+---------+---------+---------+---------+---------+---------+---------+---------+---------+

     1           ( 1)                       L.......A......H

     2           ( 0)

     3           ( 1)                                     H

     4           ( 0)

     5           ( 1)            L.............A.......H

     6           ( 1)                             H

     7           ( 1)                       H

     8           ( 1)                                     H

     9           ( 1)                                        H

    10           ( 1)                                            H

    11           ( 1)                 L......H

    12           ( 1)                                H

                              +---------+---------+---------+---------+---------+---------+---------+---------+---------+---------+
                              12400     17150     21900     26650     31400     36150     40900     45650     50400     55150     59900
```

EXHIBIT III-5

AHA Comm. Hosp. Wage/Salary Survey 3/15/xx

```
JANUARY 1981

JOB: DIR/PLANT ENGINEERING            ESTABLISHED SALARY RANGES AND ACTUAL SALARIES - BY POSITION, AND BY PARTICIPANT

                                 19000     22000     25000     28000     31000     34000     37000     40000     43000     46000     49000
PARTICIPANTS  (INCUMBENTS)       +---------+---------+---------+---------+---------+---------+---------+---------+---------+---------+

SURVEY :  1       (  1)               L............................M.......H

SURVEY :  2       (  0)

SURVEY :  3       (  1)                         L...........M....H

SURVEY :  4       (  1)                       L.....................M..........H

SURVEY :  5       (  1)                                 L.........................M.......................................H

SURVEY :  6       (  1)             L.....M...H

SURVEY :  7       (  1)                   H

                                 +---------+---------+---------+---------+---------+---------+---------+---------+---------+---------+
                                 19000     22000     25000     28000     31000     34000     37000     40000     43000     46000     49000

LEGEND :
....... ESTABLISHED SALARY RANGES
```

SECTION IV

SALARY STRUCTURE DEVELOPMENT

The salary structure is composed of monetary ranges designed to correspond to job grade levels. The salary range is created for each job grade, and all employees in a job of that grade should be compensated at levels within the salary range. Salary ranges should be developed in consideration of internal equity and rates paid for similar jobs in the market.

A. General Theory

1. Range Midpoint - Every salary range is based upon the midpoint, which should represent an externally competitive job rate for an experienced employee performing at a satisfactory level.

2. Range Spread - The size of the salary range. The room for monetary growth within the range (the range spread) varies depending on the level of the position which is designed. Range spread is usually expressed as a percentage relationship of the range maximum to the minimum. For example, a 50 % range spread indicates that the range maximum is 150% of the minimum. Salary ranges for lower level positions generally have a range spread of 25% to 30%, while the highest level positions (department heads, etc.) have salary ranges with a 50% spread.

The reason range spreads increase up the salary structure is that frequently individuals in upper level positions have much more growth potential within their existing jobs and will stay in one position for a much longer period of time than those at lower levels. At lower levels, job responsibilities are much more restricted, and an individual is more likely to receive promotions to other, higher grade levels.

3. <u>Range Minimum</u> - The range minimum should represent an externally competitive starting rate for individuals who meet the basic qualifications.

4. <u>Range Maximum</u> - The range maximum should represent the maximum amount the hospital is willing to compensate an individual for that job's contribution to the hospital's health care and delivery effort. Frequently, the upper quarter or so of the range is restricted to those individuals performing at exceptional levels.

5. <u>Midpoint Progression</u> - The midpoint progression refers to the mathematical relationship between the ranges within the structure. Since every range should be developed around the midpoint, range relationships are expressed as the percent differential between midpoints. Midpoint progressions should remain constant, or, as is most common, increase gradually up the grade structure. It is recommended that the midpoint progression not be less than 6-8%, or a meaningful difference in the compensation levels for different grades will not result. At higher grades, the midpoint progression should approximate 15% to preserve meaningful relativity of grade levels.

B. Types of Salary Structures

The type of salary structure selected should depend on the hospital's compensation policy. Sometimes, more than one type of structure may be used within an institution to deal with different groups of employees. Generally, there are three basic types of salary structures:

1. Lock-Step Structure - The lock-step structure specifies rates within the structure to be attained at designated time-in-service intervals. The structure does not recognize performance differences beyond satisfactory or unsatisfactory performance. The longevity steps are approximately 3-5% apart. Employees receive structural increases when ranges change, as well as step movements on their anniversary date. Most often, lock steps are designated at: start, six months of service, one year of service, and annually thereafter.

Sample Lock-Step Salary Range
(Applying a 4% Progression from Start)

Start	6 Mos.	1 Year	2 Years	3 Years
$4.50	$4.68	$4.87	$5.06	$5.26

Lock-step ranges are most commonly used for non-exempt positions by an institution which wishes to recognize and compensate for length of service.

Advantages of the Lock-Step Structure:

- Readily communicated and accepted by majority of employees.

- Best utilization is in organizations or for jobs where required performance standards or levels are rather tight, with little measurable latitude; or

- A rather stable work force exists, and pay rewards are justified for length of service gradations and/or to attain equity with those of less service.

- Number of steps, amount of adjustments and time spans are related to the most important organization and competitive objectives.

- Probably the most common in practice, although reluctantly admitted. Generally meets Equal Pay and EEOC requirements.

- Easy to administer by supervisors, Personnel and Payroll.

Disadvantages of Lock-Step Structure:

- Sometimes used where performance is measurable.

- No longer related to original conditions and objectives.

- Pressure for new maximum--What is the limit to rewarding longevity, per se?

- Midpoint or maximum the true competitive objective?

- Inflexible and costly, as employee generally receives two automatic increases: A) anniversary date, and B) structure movement (general).

- Difficult to manage changes.

2. Longevity/Merit Step Structure - The longevity/merit step structure is similar to the lock-step structure in design, except that movement from one step to the next is dictated by performance, rather than length of service. Frequently, high level performers move through the steps more quickly, and barely satisfactory performers move more slowly and may never reach the higher steps of the range.

Sample Longevity/Merit Step Structure

Start	6 Mos.	1 Year	2 Years	Maximum
4.50	4.68	4.87	Merit	5.26

Advantages of Longevity/Merit Step Structures:

- Readily communicated and accepted by majority of employees.

- Recognizes and rewards individual performance as well as longevity.

- Number of steps, amount of adjustments and time spans are related to most important organization and competitive objectives.

- Easy to administer by supervisors, personnel and payroll.

- Meets Equal Pay and EEOC Requirements

Disadvantages of Longevity/Merit Step Structures:

- Performance levels may not be fairly and consistently determined across departments (requires administrative control).

- Is the midpoint or maximum the true competitive rate?

- Requires the establishment and communication of effective and acceptable performance requirements.

- Applied systematically to jobs with significantly different performance requirement steps.

- Easy to abuse; frequently reduces itself to a longevity lock-step system.

3. The Open Range Structure--The Merit System - The pure merit structure consists of open ranges with a minimum, midpoint and maximum. Movement within the range is determined by performance. Established merit guidelines assure the supervision in determining the appropriateness and frequency of merit increases. Frequently, employees are reviewed for performance annually, and increases are received on an annual basis. The percentage increase received depends upon performance. In other organizations, both timing and percentage will vary according to performance.

Requirements for a Successful Merit Program

Because the foundation of a merit program is the performance appraisal process, it is essential that performance appraisals be seen as objective and equitable by employees. The best appraisal forms relate performance measurement directly to the skill and timeliness in the individual's performance of job duties, not personality characteristics. In many organizations, concrete and measurable job performance standards are developed for major job functions in order to define a job well done. In addition, all personnel with supervisory responsibilities should receive training in good performance appraisal techniques.

Sample Merit Range
(30% Spread)

Minimum	Midpoint	Maximum
$4.50	$5.17	$5.85

Sample Merit Guidelines

Performance Level	Percent Increase
Marginal	0%
Satisfactory	4 - 6%
Standard	7 - 9%
Outstanding	10 -12%

Pure merit ranges are generally used from the lowest supervisory levels through department head positions. However, many hospitals are moving to this approach for non-exempt positions as well.

Advantages of the Merit Structures:

- Directly relates pay to measurable performance on the job (a motivator).

- Perceived as fair and equitable by employees.

- Meets Equal Pay and EEOC requirements.

- Allows for flexibility in pay practices to recognize individuals in jobs.

Disadvantages of Merit Structures:

- Requires the establishment and communication of effective, acceptable and measurable performance requirements.

- Requires supervisory training in conducting effective performance appraisals.

- Performance levels may not be fairly and consistently determined across departments (requires administrative control).

- Unless structural adjustments are given when ranges are adjusted up for competitiveness, compression frequently results with the new, starting employees.

C. Sample Structural Development

AHA Community Hospital is currently on a longevity/merit step structure for non-exempt and technical positions. Supervisors and managers are on a merit structure. Once jobs have been evaluated and assigned to grades, ranges must be designed to be competitive in the external job market. The structure designer must first determine the competitiveness of existing ranges. Then, being aware of the hospital's competitive strategy, develop a new structure (or adjust the old one) for the coming year.

Exhibit IV-1 displays AHA Community's current non-exempt wage structure and Exhibit IV-2 the Supervisory/Management Salary structure.

1. Analyze Current Pay Data

a) Internal Salary Practice Line - Exhibit IV-3 displays the configuration of current average salaries by grade at AHA Community Hospital. The exhibit allows management to determine if the current internal salary practice line is competitive with external practice. Look at the average salary level for each grade and draw a line from point to point. This is the internal salary practice line.

Then, plot the external averages by grade and draw a line between the points. This is the external salary practice line.

A comparison of the two lines will indicate the degree of competitiveness of current AHA Community salaries with the external market. Looking at Exhibit IV-4, it is obvious that the March AHA Community ranges are fairly competitive with the March marketplace. However, the AHA Community pay levels look a little low in relation to the market for grades 11-17.

b) Determine Need for Adjustment - Determine how much average salaries and/or pay ranges need to go up to remain competitive in the coming year.

Exhibit IV-5 is a partial display of an analysis of current ranges and average pay levels at AHA Community and those of the external market. Looking at this exhibit, it is found that both AHA Community's ranges and average paid salaries are competitive in the higher grades of the structure. However, at lower levels, (the example is the EKG technician in grade 13), both ranges and average paid salaries appear too low.

The responses to the general questionnaire section of the external survey indicate that the competition anticipates a 9% increase in average pay levels for the coming year (See Section III). This would indicate that AHA Community must move at least this much to maintain its current competitive position.

c) Determine Competitive Position - Determine management's (or the governing body's) competitive pay strategy.

It is the desire of the Board of AHA Community to pay the "going rates" for hospital personnel; i.e., they wish AHA Community's salaries to fall approximately in the middle of the range of external salaries, or the 50th percentile of the marketplace. The board is particularly concerned about nursing pay levels, due to the shortage of nurses in the job market.

2. Construct a New Salary Structure

a) What Market Situations Need Correcting - As was discovered in Subparagraphs 1(a) and 1(b), AHA Community has fallen slightly behind current market levels in the lower grades. Through external survey analysis described in Subparagraph 1(b), it is anticipated that the average market pay levels will increase by 9% in the coming year. Exhibit IV-6 demonstrates what the anticipated external salary practice line will look like one year from now. The hospital wishes to develop a new structure that will be competitive with this next year. Obviously, ranges and salaries at lower grade levels need higher adjustments than upper levels.

b) Determine New Competitive Midpoints - Since the range midpoint should represent an externally competitive job rate for an experienced employee performing at a satisfactory level, (See Section IV-A, "General Theory") the first step in developing a new structure is to determine desirable midpoints. To correct the market situation at lower levels, these will be adjusted more than upper levels.

i) Non-Exempt Structural Adjustment - Keeping in mind that non-exempt employees receive merit step increases of approximately 6% in addition to structural adjustments, a 3% structural adjustment should be enough to maintain competitiveness of current incumbents. However, ranges should be moved more to assure competitive start rates and sufficient room for salary growth for incumbents at the higher levels of the range.

As a result, AHA Community decides to move the range midpoints from 5-7%, the 7% increase in the lower grades. This 7% increase will not immediately bring the lower grade ranges into line with the market, but should improve their position somewhat. Since AHA Community does not wish to spend all the funds necessary this year, a little more will be spent on these grades than the anticipated market movement for the next few years, so that the problem will gradually be resolved.

ii) <u>Supervisory/Management Structural Adjustment</u> - Supervisory/management employees do not receive structural adjustments at AHA Community. As a group, they receive an average merit increase of 9%. (This assumes a normal, or "bell-curve" distribution of performance ratings.) However, ranges must be adjusted up for this group for competitive start rates and reasonable room for salary growth for incumbents at the top of the range.

Since it is not anticipated that the starting salaries and average paid salaries will move up as quickly as those in lower levels, AHA Community has decided to adjust these midpoints up by 5%. See Exhibit IV-7 for the development of new midpoints. Again, the general theories regarding midpoint progression (Section IV-A) have been adhered to.

Since the existing structure range spreads proved attractive in both the bar graphs (Section III, Exhibit III-5) and in the analysis of Market Competitiveness (Exhibit IV-5 in this Section), it is determined that it is not necessary to change existing range spreads. The new minimums are checked to assure that they will be competitive in the coming year, and it appears that they will prove adequate and in line with AHA Community's competitive strategy. Based on last year's range spreads, new ranges are constructed around the midpoints. See Exhibit IV-8.

3. Estimated Cost of Recommended New Salary Structure

The final step before approval of a new structure is to develop a reasonable annual payroll cost estimate for implementation of the structure. The degree of difficulty in determining the estimate depends on how different the new structure is from the old one. If the hospital has changed from a lock-step structure to merit, or has added or deleted range steps, assumptions regarding the effect and implementation of the new structural design will have to be made to estimate the one-time cost of adopting the new design.

In the case of AHA Community Hospital, the structural adjustments do not entail dramatic changes in structural design. On the non-exempt structure, the number of steps and range spreads have remained the same. In addition, range spreads have remained the same on the supervisory/management structure. In any case, if the controller or fiscal representative is available, assistance may be sought in developing a reasonable cost estimate.

i) Structural Adjustment: Given the assumptions above, the cost of implementing the new structure (adjusting each individual to the new value of their current step in range) will be:

$3,297,000 x 106.9% = $3,524,493

or, an increase of 6.9% over current payroll. (Again, this is figured by determining the number of FTE's at each step in each grade from payroll records.)

Merit Step Adjustment - In addition, non-exempt employees at AHA Community receive step movement increases on their anniversary dates. These average 6%. Since these increases are received by employees throughout the year, the total cost will not be reflected in next year's payroll. It is a reasonable estimate to assume that an additional 4% of the new structure base cost will be incurred in the next fiscal year:

$3,524,493 x 4% = $ 140,979

Total Non-Exempt Payroll Estimate for fiscal 19X1 will be:

$3,297,000 x 111.2%= $36,666,264

or, 11.2% over last year.

ii) Determine Current Supervisory/Management Annual Payroll - The current supervisory/management annual payroll at CSI Community is:

$1,413,000

As stated in "Hospital Policy," there are no structural adjustments for employees on the supervisory/management structure. Again, merit increases occur throughout the year on employee service dates, so that the full average increase of 9% will not be incurred during the fiscal year. It is estimated that three quarters of this, or 6.75% of current payroll, will be incurred in the fiscal year.

$1,413,000 x 6.75% = $ **95,378**

or, annual payroll for new supervisory/management structure of:

$1,508,378

iii) Total Annual Payroll Costs

	Existing Structures	Recommended Structures
N-E	$3,297,000	$3,665,472
S/M	1,413,000	1,508,378
TOTAL	$4,710,000	$5,173,850

TOTAL PERCENTAGE CHANGE: 9.8%

NOTE: Cost estimates are only estimates, and should be treated as such. Check validity of assumptions by checking past payroll history.

4. Submit Recommended Structures - Submit recommended structures and cost estimates for necessary approvals. Many hospitals have a compensation committee composed of the personnel representative, the Chief Administrator and some members of the governing body. Decisions regarding implementation procedures for adoption of the new structure (See Section V.) should also be made with this group.

EXHIBIT IV-1

AHA COMMUNITY HOSPITAL

NON-EXEMPT WAGE STRUCTURE

OCTOBER 1, 19XX

MIDPOINT PROGRESSION	GRADE	START	SIX MONTHS	MERIT STEP	MIDPOINT (JOB RATE) MERIT STEP	MERIT STEP	RANGE SPREAD
	11	$3.35	$3.60	$3.85	$4.11	$4.36	30%
7%	12	3.58	3.85	4.12	4.36	4.60	30%
8%	13	3.87	4.16	4.45	4.74	5.03	30%
9%	14	4.21	4.53	4.84	5.16	5.48	30%
10%	15	4.63	4.98	5.33	5.68	6.02	30%
11%	16	5.06	5.47	5.88	6.28	6.68	32%
12%	17	5.67	6.13	6.58	7.03	7.48	32%
12%	18	6.27	6.82	7.37	7.92	8.46	35%

AHA COMMUNITY HOSPITAL

SUPERVISORY/MANAGEMENT SALARY STRUCTURE

OCTOBER 1, 19XX

GRADE	MIDPOINT PROGRESSION	MINIMUM	MIDPOINT	MAXIMUM	RANGE SPREAD
A		13,770	16,524	19,278	40%
	12%				
B		15,385	18,462	21,539	40%
	12%				
C		16,879	20,677	24,475	45%
	13%				
D		18,720	23,400	28,080	50%
	15%				
E		21,520	26,900	32,280	50%

EXHIBIT IV-3

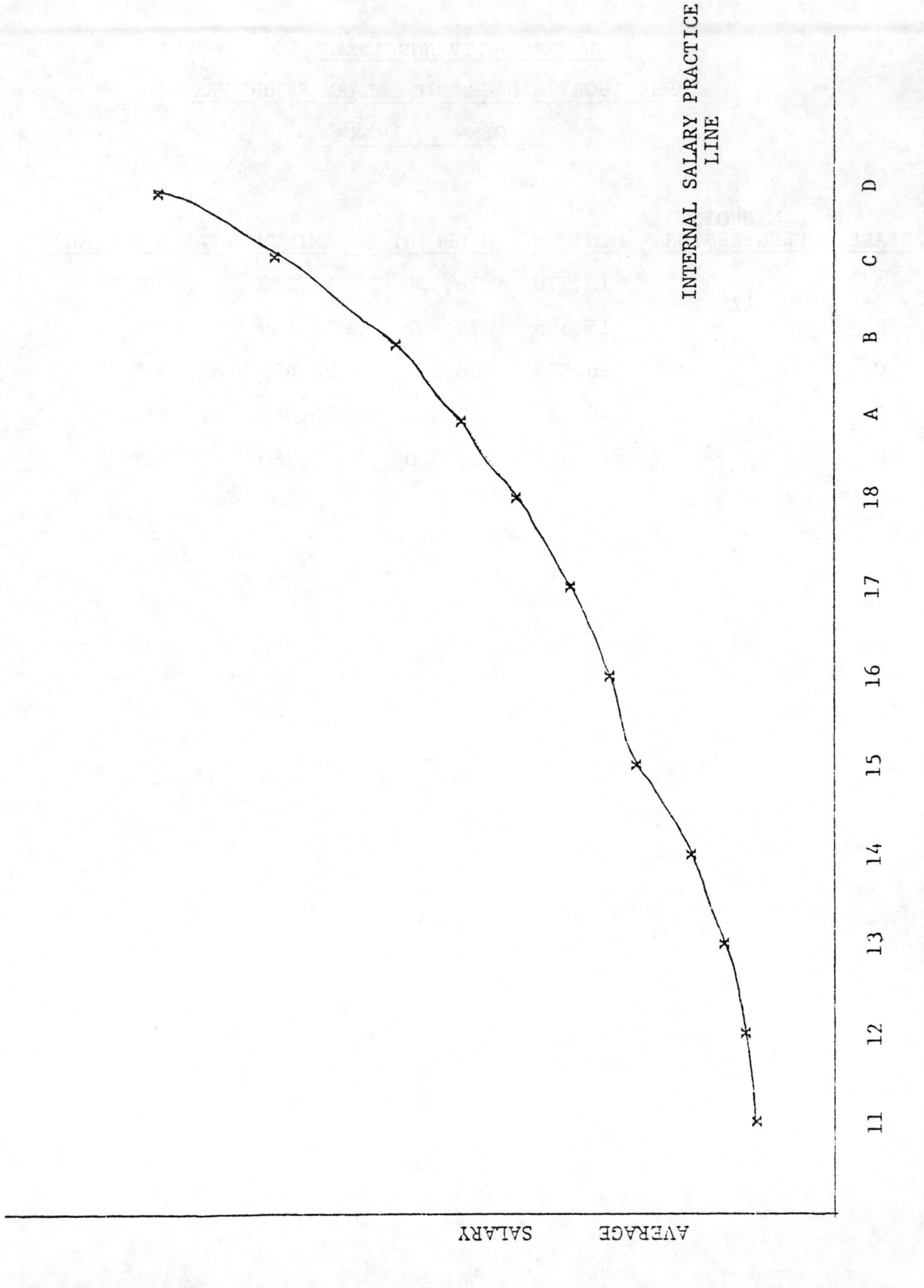

INTERNAL SALARY PRACTICE LINE

AVERAGE SALARY

11 12 13 14 15 16 17 18 A B C D

EXHIBIT IV-4

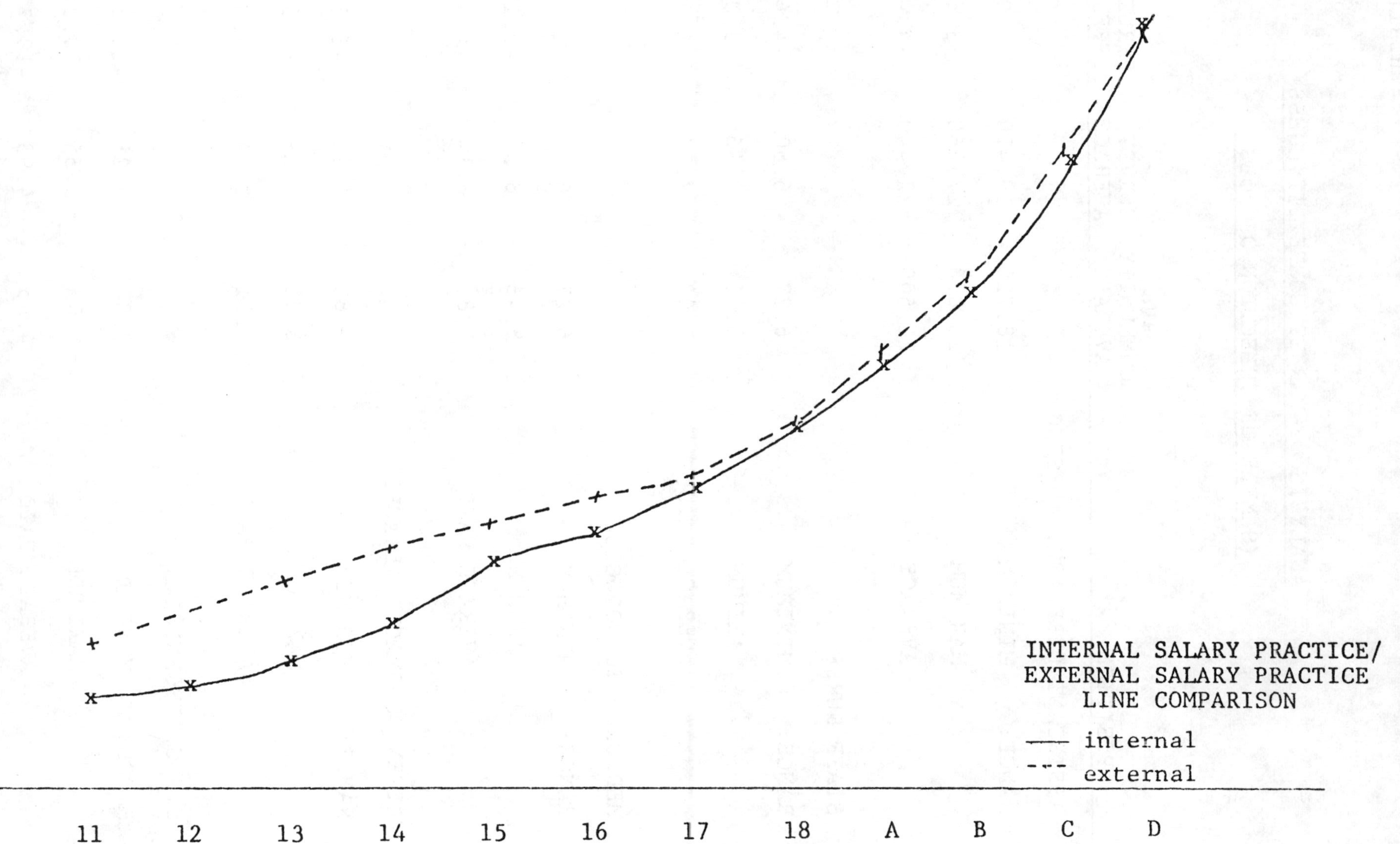
INTERNAL SALARY PRACTICE/
EXTERNAL SALARY PRACTICE
LINE COMPARISON
internal
external
AVERAGE SALARY
11
12
13
14
15
16
17
18
A
B
C
D

EXHIBIT IV-5

ANALYSIS OF MARKET COMPETITIVENESS

(SAMPLE OF SELECTION OF JOBS)

GRADE	POSITION		AHA COMMUNITY AVERAGE	SURVEY AVERAGE	PERCENT DIFFERENCE	COMMENTS
D	ASSISTANT DIRECTOR, NURSING					
	RANGE:	MINIMUM	18,720	19,470	-4.0%	RANGE AND AVERAGE PAID COMPETITIVE (SLIGHTLY LOW)
		MAXIMUM	28,080	27,060	+3.6%	
		AVERAGE PAID	21,500	22,440	-4.4%	
18	STAFF NURSE					
	RANGE:	MINIMUM	6.27	6.50	-4.4%	STARTING SALARY LOW RANGE IN GENERAL, AVERAGE PAID COMPETITIVE
		MAXIMUM	8.46	8.46	0.0%	
		AVERAGE PAID	7.03	7.12	-1.3%	
18	MEDICAL TECHNOLOGIST					
	RANGE:	MINIMUM	6.27	6.40	-2.1%	
		MAXIMUM	8.46	8.51	-0.1%	
		AVERAGE PAID	7.80	8.14	-4.4%	
15	LICENSED PRACTICAL NURSE					
	RANGE:	MINIMUM	4.63	4.92	-6.3%	
		MAXIMUM	6.02	6.29	-4.5%	
		AVERAGE PAID	5.21	5.44	-4.4%	
13	E.K.G. TECHNICIAN					
	RANGE:	MINIMUM	3.87	4.28	-10.5%	
		MAXIMUM	5.03	5.55	-10.3%	
		AVERAGE PAID	4.45	4.93	-10.7%	

EXHIBIT IV-6

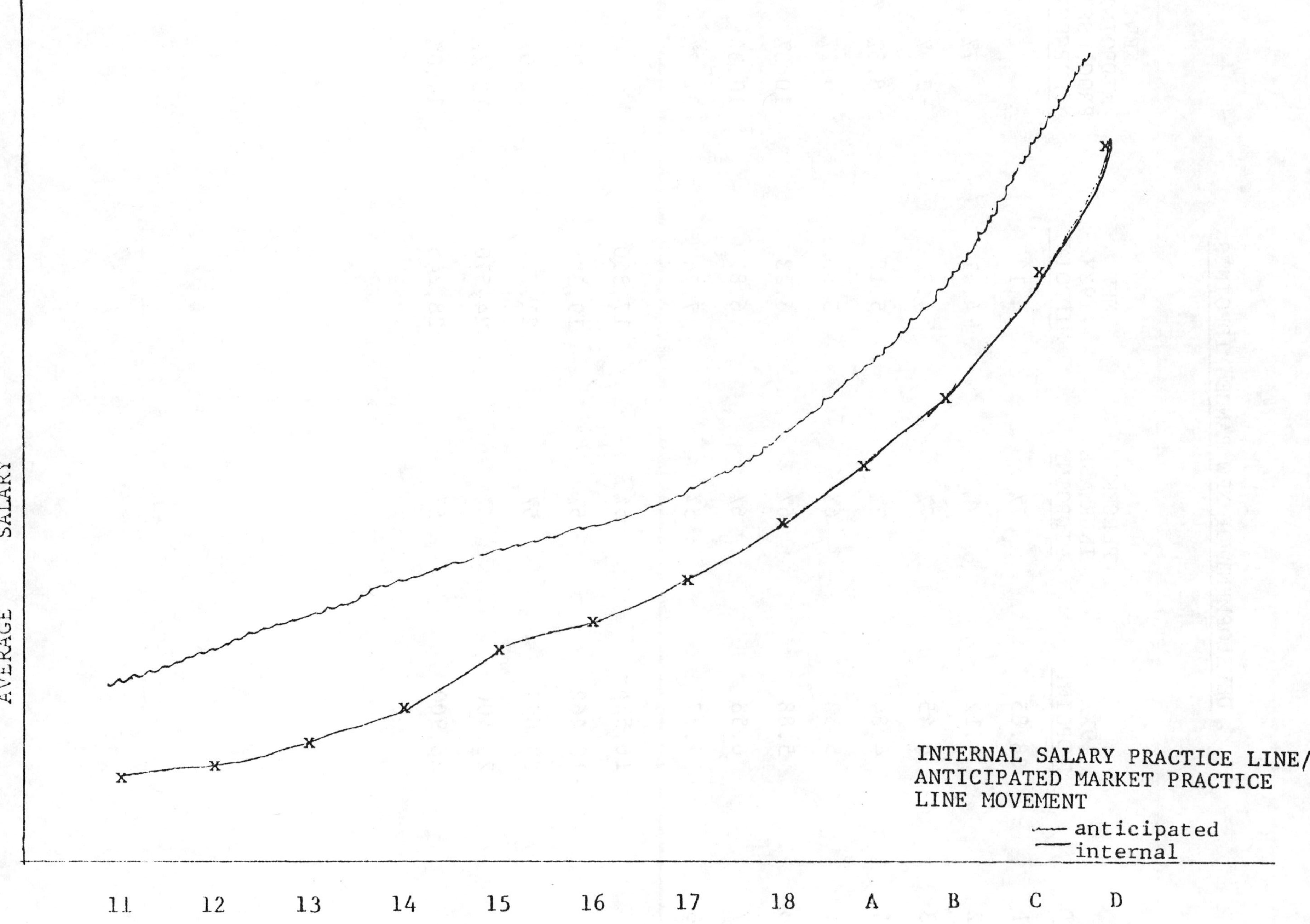

AVERAGE SALARY
INTERNAL SALARY PRACTICE LINE/
ANTICIPATED MARKET PRACTICE
LINE MOVEMENT
anticipated
internal
11
12
13
14
15
16
17
18
A
B
C
D

DEVELOPMENT OF NEW RANGE MIDPOINTS

GRADE	19XX MIDPOINT	PERCENT INCREASE MIDPOINT	NEW 19XX MIDPOINT	NEW MIDPOINT PROGRESSION (PERCENT)
11	$3.85	7%	4.12	
12	4.12	7%	4.41	7%
13	4.45	7%	4.76	7.9%
14	4.84	7%	5.18	8.8%
15	5.33	6%	5.65	9.1%
16	5.88	6%	6.23	10.3%
17	6.58	6%	6.87	10.3%
18	7.37	5%	7.74	12.7%
A	16,524	5%	17,350	
B	18,462	5%	19,385	11.7%
C	20,677	5%	21,711	12,0%
D	23,400	5%	24,570	13.2%
E	26,900	5%	28,245	14.0%

CONSTRUCTION OF NEW RANGES AROUND MIDPOINTS

NON-EXEMPT STRUCTURE

GRADE	MINIMUM (START)	SIX * MONTHS	MIDPOINT MERIT STEP	MERIT STEP*	MERIT STEP	RANGE STEP PERCENT
11	3.58	3.85	4.12	4.36	4.66	30%
12	3.84	4.13	4.41	4.70	4.98	30%
13	4.14	4.45	4.76	5.07	5.38	30%
14	4.51	4.85	5.18	5.52	5.86	30%
15	4.92	5.29	5.65	6.02	6.39	30%
16	5.36	5.80	6.23	6.65	7.07	32%
17	5.92	6.40	6.87	7.34	7.81	32%
18	6.58	7.16	7.74	8.31	8.88	35%

* These steps are computed here as the midpoint between adjacent steps. They may also be computed as a percentage increase over the preceeding step.

HELPFUL HINT: RANGE SPREAD CORRESPONDS TO THE RELATIONSHIP OF THE MINIMUM TO THE MIDPOINT. THE FOLLOWING TABLE MAY ASSIST IN DEVELOPING RANGES AROUND THE MIDPOINT.

FOR THIS RANGE SPREAD	MINIMUM IS THIS % OF MIDPOINT
25%	= 89%
27%	= 88%
30%	= 87%
32%	= 86%
35%	= 85%
40%	= 83.3%
45%	= 81.6%
50%	= 80%

CONSTRUCTION OF NEW RANGES AROUND MIDPOINTS

SUPERVISORY/MANAGEMENT STRUCTURE

GRADE	MINIMUM	MIDPOINT	MAXIMUM	RANGE SPREAD
A	$14,458	17,350	20,241	40
B	16,154	19,385	22,615	40
C	7,723	21,711	25,698	45
D	19,656	24,570	29,484	50
E	22,596	28,245	33,894	50

SECTION V

IMPLEMENTATION OF A NEW SALARY STRUCTURE

Once a new salary structure and/or program has received the necessary approvals, a concrete implementation plan must be developed to assure a smooth transition. Obviously, the magnitude of the change will determine the difficulty of the implementation process.

A. Exceptions to the New Program

If the salary program is changing dramatically, it is not reasonable to expect to have all salaries in line with the new structure(s) in the first year. If the hospital has not historically had a comprehensive compensation program, the job evaluation and market analysis processes may significantly alter existing relativities in the organization. For this reason, current incumbent salaries may be out of line with the new grade and salary structure.

Three problem salary situations develop in adopting a new structure:

1. Green Circles: Those employees whose salaries fall below the minimum of their newly created range. Generally, their salaries are brought up to the new minimum at the time of the structural change, unless the cost is prohibitive, or the amount needed to reach the minimum is so significant it is done in phased steps. However, it is recommended that all salaries attain range minimums within one year of the structure implementation.

2. <u>Red Circles</u>: Those employees whose salaries are above the maximum of their newly created range. For employee relations reasons, these individuals rarely have their salaries reduced. Hospital management makes the decision to either freeze their salaries until successive structure adjustments over the years bring the range in line with their salaries, or give the individuals increases smaller than the annual structural adjustments so that over a period of time, their ranges and salaries gradually fall in line. Most frequently, the latter alternative is selected. Though this alternative assures that it will take longer for the ranges and salaries to fall in line, hospital management does not wish to "penalize" incumbents by the adoption of a new wage and salary program. It assists the management effort in gaining acceptance of the new program.

3. <u>Orange Circles</u>: Those employees whose salaries, on a step structure, fall into an inappropriate place within the range according to program guidelines. For example, suppose at AHA Community a job on the non-exempt structure is downgraded. The current incumbent's salary is within the range, but is too high, based on his performance and longevity, relative to the other employees already in the lower grade. This is an orange circle employee. As in the case of the red circles above, the employee is rarely "penalized" for organizational changes, but his salary is gradually phased into the program over a period of time.

When the evaluation program, or the timing or number of steps in a step program, is altered, orange circle situations frequently develop. The most important thing is to develop a plan to deal with these people fairly and consistently. What is done depends largely on the funds the hospital has available, the management philosophy of the hosptial, and the current employee relations climate.

B. Development of Salary Administration Manual

A detailed formal statement of policies and procedures for the salary administration program should be written and distributed to supervisors and managers to assure equitable and consistent application of the program across all departments in the hospital.

The manual should include policies and procedures on the following:

- Hiring and/or starting salary policies.

- How to determine increases for individual employees.

- Job description procedures.

- How to apply for re-evaluation of a position.

- Promotion, transfer and demotion policies.

- How to apply for exceptional salary treatment for an individual.

- Definitions of the levels of authority of supervisors, managers, department heads, personnel and administration.

- Merit guidelines and performance appraisal procedures (if on a merit program).

The manual should also reiterate the goals and philosophies of the program, and access to the manual should be limited to those employees with supervisory responsibilities. Sample forms (job questionnaires, performance appraisal forms, recommendation for salary increase forms, etc.,) may also be included.

C. Training Supervisors and Managers in the New Program

Supervisors and managers must be trained in the new program's policies and procedures. It is important that they understand and support the philosophies underlying the program so that they are communicated properly to their employees. Using the manual described in the previous section, the trainer should be sure supervisors understand all the policies and procedures therein.

In merit systems, the supervisors and managers must be trained in performance appraisal techniques and procedures, as the equity and success of the program depends upon the meaningfulness and objectivity of the performance review.

D. Communication of the Salary Administration Program

In addition to the supervisory training discussed in the previous section, the philosophies and goals of the compensation program should be communicated to the Board of Directors, Department Heads and all employees. Frequently, a formal statement of policies and goals, such as is seen in Section I, is included in an announcement to all employees, whether it is in the in-house publication or in a special letter distributed to employees. Such an announcement should come from the Chief Administrator, demonstrating his belief and support of the new program. See Exhibit V-3 for a sample announcement. Frequently, too, Evaluation Committee members are ready and willing to serve as effective advocates of the new program.

The amount of information regarding the program given to employees depends largely on the style of management at the hospital. To assure employee acceptance, however, a brief outline of the program should be explained. At a minimum, the employee should know the following things:

- Current salary.

- Current job grade.

- Date of next salary review.

- What salary increases are dependent upon (performance and/or longevity).

- That a job evaluation system exists.

- The hospital's goals in the compensation program.

- How they will be affected by the new program.

Some hospitals briefly explain the job evaluation plan factors and the Committee process; others do not (though supervisory and management personnel are informed). Frequently, too, hospital management tells their employees that a goal of their program is to remain competitive with other area employers, but believe it is inappropriate to detail the competitive strategy of the institution.

E. Ongoing Administration of the Salary Administration Program

It is important to note that development of wage and salary programs is a continuous process, and is not "finished" with the completion of job evaluations and the adoption of a new salary structure. Jobs in the health care field are constantly changing, as are organizations. Consequently, hospital positions must be periodically reviewed and redefined. The changes may cause a re-evaluation and result in job up-grading or down-grading. In addition, external market rates for health care positions are continually moving in response to inflation and supply and demand. Therefore, it is essential to continually monitor internal and external changes to fulfill program goals of internal equity and external competitiveness. The program administrator must not hesitate to make revisions as required, following sound compensation principles.

Schedule for ongoing compensation program maintenance:

To assure that the compensation program continues to remain sound, all tools and methodologies should be periodically reviewed by top Administration personnel.

Statutory Considerations:

An assigned individual should keep abreast of regulatory changes affecting compensation programs, and assure the hospital that all aspects of the hospital's compensation program remain in compliance.

Job Descriptions: The personnel representative should be assigned the responsibility of a schedule to audit all job descriptions at least once every two years, to be sure they are accurate and up-to-date. In addition to the audit function, this individual should assure the hospital that job descriptions are revised, as job functions change on a continual basis.

Job Evaluation: Jobs should be evaluated when they change significantly enough to require description revision. As a result, the Job Evaluation Committee is a standing committee, usually meeting once a month to review and evaluate any revised or new job descriptions.

Market Surveys: Market surveys should be done on an "as needed" basis, but at least once a year to assure that hospital wage rates continue to be competitive in the job market. This will also enable the hospital to estimate future job market behavior to revise current pay structures.

Structure Revision: In most hospitals, pay structures are revised one a year and implemented at the beginning of the new fiscal year.

A typical annual schedule for these activities, assuming a January-to-January payroll year, follows:

Activity	Timing of Activity
Incorporating statutory guideline changes	Ongoing; as they occur
Job description revision	Ongoing; as job changes occur
Job evaluation	Ongoing; as job changes develop
Special need surveys	As required
Annual survey	August-September
Revised structure design and costing	September-October
Management approval of structure revisions and related policies	October
Payroll budget development	October-December
Revised structure implementation	January 1

Adherence to a schedule of monitoring and reviewing the compensation program prevents the need for major time-consuming overhauls to bring the program back into line with hospital management's goals and objectives and market place forces. It is recommended that a specific position on the Administrative (or Personnel) Staff be assigned these responsibilities.

EXHIBIT V-1

SAMPLE

PRESENTATION TO THE BOARD INFORMING THEM OF THE DEVELOPMENT OF A COMPENSATION PROGRAM

As you are aware, AHA Community Hospital is currently spending $4.7 million on our personnel payroll. We have decided to undertake a thorough study of internal and external compensation practice, with the following goals:

1. To fairly compensate employees for work performed in comparison to other positions in the Hospital.

2. To compensate employees at levels competitive with the external market.

3. To recognize and reward longevity and performance.

To attain these goals, we will be performing the following steps:

A. All jobs will be thoroughly documented and job descriptions written by the first-line supervisors and approved by department heads.

B. All jobs will be evaluated by a committee of department heads using a point-factor job evaluation plan. This is a process of measuring each job against ten compensable factors.

   1) Mental Development - the developed intellectual capacity necessary to apply the skills required by the job requirements.

2) Work Experience - the amount and level of experience on the job or in directly related work needed by the average employee with the specified level of mental development to gain the skills required to perform work of acceptable quality and quantity.

3) Judgment - the mental ability, ingenuity and job knowledge required to relate business, scientific or craft variables to policy and procedure decisions.

4) Errors and Losses - the effects of employee errors.

5) Resource Utilization - the responsibility to effectively and efficiently employ the resources of the Hospital.

6) Systems and Data - responsibility to help the processes and systems of the Hospital in operation.

7) Interpersonal Relationships - the frequency and depth of job relationships with other departments in the Hospital.

8) Work Environment - the elements of work surroundings or work schedules that tend to be disagreeable.

9) Hazards - inherent job conditions which potentially endanger the safety and health of the incumbent.

10) Personal Demands - the physical and mental demands of the position.

The completion of Steps A and B should move us toward fulfillment of Goal #1.

C. Next, Personnel will survey pay levels for similar jobs at other hospitals (Goal #2).

D. Personnel will design a pay structure incorporating the internal and external results to create a pay system which is internally equitable and externally competitive.

E. We will plan how to implement and administer the pay system on this structure to recognize individual longevity and performance, as we have in the past.

F. We will cost the new program and come to you for approval. We anticipate, however, that the cost will involve an increase of two percent of current payroll (in addition to normal pay structure increase costs) to correct some internal inequities.

In all, we anticipate the project will be completed in one year. We in Administration feel very strongly that this project is necessary. With rapidly increasing payroll costs, we must have a compensation program that effectively allocates limited payroll funds. In addition, guidelines from the EEOC and other regulatory agencies require that we have a coherent, defensible pay program.

With your approval, we would like to announce the project and get started. In order for this to be successful, we must have your strong support, for this will involve a lot of effort on the part of many of our employees.

EXHIBIT V-2

SAMPLE

PRESENTATION TO THE DEPARTMENT HEADS INFORMING THEM OF THE DEVELOPMENT OF A COMPENSATION PROGRAM

I am pleased to announce that AHA Community Hospital will be undertaking a thorough study of our compensation program. It will involve quite a bit of work on all our parts, but it will be time well spent. Because of increasing payroll costs, a rapidly fluctuating job market, recent EEO and governmental guidelines, and increased employee awareness, we must have a systematic, defensible compensation program.

The goals of this program are:

1. To fairly compensate employees for work performed in comparison to other positions in the Hospital.

2. To compensate employees at levels competitive with the external market.

3. To recognize and reward longevity and performance.

To attain these goals, we will be performing the following steps:

A. All jobs will be thoroughly documented and job descriptions written by the first-line supervisors and approved by department heads.

   We realize that this will take a lot of time for all of you, but it is essential that we have complete, accurate job descriptions to conduct the rest of the project, as you can see from the following steps.

B. All jobs will be evaluated by a committee of department heads using a point-factor job evaluation plan. This is a process of measuring each job against ten compensable factors.

1) Mental Development - the developed intellectual capacity necessary to apply the skills required by the job requirements.

   If you wish to be a part of this committee, please see me after the meeting. While it involves a big time commitment, it will be a very interesting experience for everyone involved. It is a one-of-a-kind opportunity to learn what functions are performed in other departments. We will be selecting a committee to assure representation from as many areas of the Hospital as possible.

2) Work Experience - the amount and level of experience on the job or in directly related work needed by the average employee with the specified level of mental development to gain the skills required to perform work of acceptable quality and quantity.

3) Judgment - the mental ability, ingenuity and job knowledge required to relate business, scientific or craft variables to policy and procedure decisions.

4) Errors and Losses - the effects of employee errors.

5) Resource Utilization - the responsibility to effectively and efficiently employ the resources of the Hospital.

6) Systems and Data - responsibility to help the processes and systems of the Hospital in operation.

7) Interpersonal Relationships - the frequency and depth of job relationships with other departments in the Hospital.

8) Work Environment - the elements of work surroundings or work schedules that tend to be disagreeable.

9) Hazards - inherent job conditions which potentially endanger the safety and health of the incumbent.

10) Personal Demands - the physical and mental demands of the position.

The completion of Steps A and B should fulfill Goal #1.

C. Next, Personnel will survey pay levels for similar jobs at other hospitals (Goal #2).

D. Personnel will design a pay structure incorporating the internal and external results to create a pay system which is internally equitable and externally competitive.

E. We will plan how to implement and administer the pay system on this structure to recognize individual longevity and performance, as we have in the past.

In all, we anticipate the project will be completed in one year. We in Administration feel very strongly that this project is necessary. With rapidly increasing payroll costs, we must have a compensation program that effectively allocates limited payroll funds. In addition, guidelines from the EEOC and other regulatory agencies require that we have a coherent, defensible pay program.

SAMPLE PRESENTATION TO THE EMPLOYEES INFORMING THEM OF THE NEW COMPENSATION PROGRAM

NEW SALARY PROGRAM!

AHA Community Hospital is pleased to announce the implementation of an entirely new wage and salary system for our employees. For some time, the hospital has been aware of the need for improved competitiveness in our compensation, for increased equitability in the pay given each position in the hospital, and above all, of the need for a pay system which recognizes both performance and time of service. We are delighted that such a program is now in place.

Over the past few months, the administration has been working to determine the best possible approach to compensation. We have conducted extensive wage and salary surveys with nearby hospitals similar to ours to determine the "market value" of existing positions, and to assure that our pay levels are competitive with those offered by other hospitals. We have analyzed our job descriptions (using information from staff) and have used an objective system for "job evaluation" to determine the relative position which each job should hold in our salary structure. We also have statistically analyzed our salary grades and ranges to make certain that each person has the opportunity to advance equitably within his or her salary level, and that each level is properly related to the other.

Finally, the administration has developed a merit system which takes into account both job performance and the amount of time an employee has been on the staff at AHA Community Hospital. Again, the ultimate goal has been to develop a pay system which both motivates employees to give their best efforts, and rewards their long-term loyalty.

Naturally, the implementation of such a plan will impact the salaries of many employees here. Assurances have been given, however, that no one will have his or her pay reduced as a result of the study; however, many people will receive unscheduled pay increases--another piece of good news! Your supervisor will be contacting you soon to tell you specifically what impact the new system will have on you.

APPENDIX A

POINT FACTOR

JOB EVALUATION PLAN

FOR

HOSPITAL POSITIONS

APPENDIX A

POINT FACTOR JOB EVALUATION PLAN FOR HOSPITAL POSITIONS

TABLE OF CONTENTS

I. Evaluation Plan Overview

I. Evaluation Plan Overview

The point factor job evaluation plan for hospital positions measures job content in terms of skill, responsibility, working conditions and effort. There are ten factors in the plan, as follows:

SKILL

The skill factors measure the knowledge required and its use in performing the job. The skill factors are:

Factor 1 - Mental Development - Mental Development refers to the developed intellectual capacity necessary to acquire and apply the skills required by the job. It is measured in terms of the prerequisite job requirements, rather than in terms of formal education.

Factor 2 - Work Experience - Work Experience refers to the amount and level of experience on the job or in directly related work required for the average ~~inexperienced~~ worker with the specified mental development to be able to perform work of acceptable quality and quantity.

Factor 3 - Judgment - Judgment refers to the mental ability, ingenuity and job knowledge required to relate business, scientific or craft variables to policy and procedure decisions, work methods, interpersonal contacts, etc., without recourse to supervision.

RESPONSIBILITY

The responsibility factors measure the accountability for accomplishing specific tasks and for care of hospital facilities, equipment, records, etc. The responsibility factors are:

Factor 4 - Errors and Losses - Errors and Losses refers to the opportunity for and consequences resulting from failure to properly perform the duties of the job. Errors affect patient care and well-being, safety of other employees or hospital reputation.

Factor 5 - Resource Utilization - Resource Utilization refers to the responsibility to effectively employ the resources of the hospital - facilities, equipment, personnel, financial.

Factor 6 - Systems and Data - Systems and Data refers to the responsibility to keep the processes and systems of the hospital in operation, on schedule and secure. This includes responsibility to work as a team member and to maintain confidentiality of business and patient information, such as medical records, test reports, employee salaries, budgets, costs, etc.

Factor 7 - Interpersonal Relationships - Interpersonal Relationships refers to the responsibility for instruction, supervision and contacts with hospital employees, patients or outside agencies.

WORKING CONDITIONS

The work condition factors measure the effects of job environment and inherent hazards. The working condition factors are:

Factor 8 - Work Environment - Work Environment refers to the elements of work, surroundings or work schedules which tend to be disagreeable or make the work more difficult.

Factor 9 - Hazards - Hazards refers to inherent job conditions which potentially endanger the health and safety of the job incumbent, such as radiation, patient behavior, stress situations, moving machinery, etc.

EFFORT

The effort factor measures mental and physical effort required by the job. The effort factor is:

Factor 10 - Personal Demands - Personal Demands refers to the physical demands, such as awkward positions, heavy lifting, etc., and the mental demands, such as concentration, attention, perception, etc.

II. Point Values

II. Point Values

	Point Value		
	Minimum		Maximum
SKILL (40-200)			
1. MENTAL DEVELOPMENT	15	-	75
2. WORK EXPERIENCE	15	-	75
3. JUDGMENT	10	-	50
RESPONSIBILITY (45-225)			
4. ERRORS AND LOSSES	10	-	50
5. RESOURCE UTILIZATION	10	-	50
6. SYSTEMS AND DATA	10	-	50
7. INTERPERSONAL RELATIONSHIPS	15	-	75
WORKING CONDITIONS (10-50)			
8. WORK ENVIRONMENT	5	-	25
9. HAZARDS	5	-	25
EFFORT (10-50)			
10. PERSONAL DEMANDS	10	-	50

III. Evaluation Factors

FACTOR #1

MENTAL DEVELOPMENT

Mental Development refers to the developed intellectual capacity necessary to apply the skills required by the job. It is measured in terms of prerequisite job requirements, rather than in terms of education.

The maximum requirements constituting a recurring part of the job determines the degree to be assigned. Emergency work or infrequent assistance to another employee are not considered.

Degree	Definition	Points
1.	General knowledge of language usage, arithmetic and/or basic science.	15
2.	General knowledge of language usage, arithmetic and/or basic science; general knowledge of the basics in a specialized occupational field.	30
3.	General knowledge of language usage, mathematics and/or scientific principles. Specific knowledge of the basic job requirements and their application in a specialized occupational field.	45

Factor #1

Mental Development (Continued)

Degree	Definition	Points
4.	Specific knowledge of language usage, mathematics and/or scientific principles; specific knowledge of the principles of a recognized field of learning and of their application in a specialized occupational field.	60
5.	Specific knowledge of language usage, mathematics and/or scientific principles; detailed specific knowledge of the background and principles of a recognized field of learning and of their application in a specialized occupational field.	75

FACTOR #2

WORK EXPERIENCE

Work Experience refers to the amount and level of experience on the job or on directly related work required for the average, inexperienced employee with the specified level of mental development to gain the skills required to perform work of acceptable quality and quantity.

Evaluation should be based on continuous progress. Assign the degree which reflects the total Work Experience to learn all phases of the job. Emergency work or infrequent assistance to another employee not normally a part of the job are not to be considered.

Degree	Definition	Points
1.	Previous experience is not required. Only normal indoctrination in job routine is necessary.	15
2.	Orientation and basic on-the-job training is required to learn job routines and work layout.	30
3.	Proficiency in entry level job and extensive on-the-job training is required to learn policies, procedures and job routines.	45
4.	Proficiency in more than one level of entry job, supervision of lower level work or proficiency in more than one specialty within an occupational field is required.	60

Factor #2

Work Experience (Continued)

Degree	Definition	Points
5.	Proficiency in all aspects of an occupational field, management of the overall function and continuing work experience to stay abreast of a continually changing job is required.	75

FACTOR #3

JUDGMENT

Judgment refers to the mental ability, ingenuity and job knowledge required to relate business, scientific or craft variables to policy and procedure decisions, work methods, interpersonal contacts, etc., without recourse to supervision.

The maximum requirements which are a normal and recurring part of the job determine the degree to be assigned.

Degree	Definition	Points
1.	Simple, routine work with little complexity; limited variations in job routines and instructions.	10
2.	Work from detailed job procedures or instructions with some room for judgment in routine; limited follow-up responsibility.	20
3.	Work follows professional, business or operation standard practice for the job; within standard practice, judgment is required to solve specific job problems from time to time.	30
4.	Work generally follows professional, business or operation standard practice, but may require deviations; majority of time is spent in problem solving or decision-making.	40

Factor #3

Judgment (Continued)

Degree	Definition	Points
5.	Work frequently deviates from standard professional, business or operation practice, requiring research, experimentation or negotiation to do the job; major problem solving and decision making responsibilities are involved.	50

FACTOR #4

ERRORS AND LOSSES

Responsibility for errors and losses refers to the effects of employee error in such things as interpreting instruction, reading labels or instruments, maintaining records or accounts, installing equipment, etc., and resulting effect (losses) on patient care, hospital facilities or equipment, safety of others, hospital records, etc.

Care required to avoid the error and loss that might result from a single error should be considered to determine the degree level.

Degree	Definition	Points
1.	Minor responsibility for errors or losses; supervisor is assigned responsibility for errors and losses.	10
2.	Normal care required to avoid error and prevent loss; close review of work by others; e.g., may be responsible for minor patient care, small amounts of cash or simple machines.	20
3.	Considerable care required to prevent errors and losses; only general review of work by others; e.g., patient care depends on data; payment of improper charges; exposure of others to significant, though not lost-time, injury.	30

Factor #4

Errors and Losses (Continued)

Degree	Definition	Points
4.	Constant care required to detailed or complex job functions or routines; only general review of work by others, generally after action is taken; e.g., administering drugs; reporting hospital compliance with complex regulations, testing or repairing major electrical systems; exposure of others to lost-time injury.	40
5.	Extreme care required in detailed or complex job routines; little opportunity to check work before effects; losses might involve patients' or employees' lives or hospital's reputation.	50

FACTOR #5
RESOURCE UTILIZATION

Resource utilization refers to the responsibility to effectively and efficiently employ the resources of the hospital--facilities, equipment, materials, personnel, financial.

Resource utilization is measured by considering both the total resources and the degree of control over those resources.

Degree	Definition	Points
1.	Little responsibility beyond the use of own time and limited working materials.	10
2.	Actions may affect utilization of co-workers; uses office machines, power tools, monitors, etc., which require planning and care for efficient operation; prepares reports, etc., which have impact on hospital finances; controls materials in use.	20
3.	Responsible for effective and efficient utilization of the resources of a section or group; prepares or is responsible for reports, etc., which if improperly done, would have a significant impact; controls ordering, receipt and stocking of materials; responsibility for utilization of major equipment systems.	30

Factor #5

Resource Utilization (Continued)

Degree	Definition	Points
4.	Responsible for effective and efficient utilization of the resources of a department; prepares or is responsible for preparation of reports, billings, payments, etc., which if improperly done, would have a significant and lasting impact on hospital finances and would require corrective action; responsibility for developing specifications, purchasing and utilizing major facilities or equipment.	40
5.	Responsible for effective and efficient utilization of the resources of a division made up of more than one department; controls a significant part of the resources of the hospital.	50

FACTOR #6

SYSTEMS AND DATA

Responsibility for systems and data refers to the job requirements for activity to keep the processes and systems of the hospital in operation, on schedule and secure. This includes responsibility to work as a member of a team and to maintain confidentiality of medical or business data.

Degree	Definition	Points
1.	Limited responsibility for systems and data; effects generally limited to use of own time.	10
2.	Work as part of a team where others are able to keep system or process going with sub-standard input or to handle data which requires some discretion.	20
3.	Work as part of a team where others are not able to make up for sub-standard performance, but which is not critical to the functioning of the hospital, or regularly handles restricted information or data, or shares responsibility for a process needed for hospital operation.	30

Factor #6

Systems and Data (Continued)

Degree	Definition	Points
4.	Responsibility for a system or process where sub-standard performance causes serious consequences for a significant sub-division of the hospital, or work with data which, if revealed, could cause serious embarrassment to the hospital or responsibility for a process needed for hospital operation.	40
5.	Responsibility for a system or process where sub-standard performance poses serious consequences for the entire hospital or work with data which, if revealed, could have serious legal or professional implications.	50

FACTOR #7
INTERPERSONAL RELATIONSHIPS

Interpersonal relationships refers to the responsibility for instruction and leadership, and to contacts with patients, the public, outside agencies, and hospital employees. These are responsibilities which must be executed effectively in order for others to properly do their jobs, or for the hospital to provide quality, efficient and courteous medical care.

Degree	Definition	Points
1.	Leadership or contact responsibility is limited to assisting others in their functions or working with new employees.	15
2.	Leadership limited to making daily work assignments or carrying out projects, or regular and substantive contact with other departments; occasional, but limited, outside contacts.	30
3.	Supervisory responsibility, including instruction and leadership, over a section or small department; and/or frequent and substantive contacts with patients, visitors, other departments, outside agencies, etc., where contacts are made within context of standard procedures or practices.	45

Factor #7

Interpersonal Relationships (Continued)

Degree	Definition	Points
4.	Responsibility for a department or small division doing highly diversified or technical work, and/or regular contact with patients, doctors, visitors or outside agencies in difficult and disturbing situations.	60
5.	Managerial responsibility for a division of more than one department doing diversified or technical work or professional level teaching or outside contacts not covered by policy or procedure requiring persuasion of others in difficult and significant matters.	75

FACTOR #8

WORK ENVIRONMENT

Work environment refers to the elements of work, surroundings or work schedules which tend to be disagreeable or to make the work more difficult. These include, but are not limited to: dust, oil, fumes, water, heat, cold, vibrations, noise, dirt.

The average working conditions on a year-round basis determine the degree to be selected.

Degree	Definition	Points
1.	Disagreeable elements are negligible. Good light and ventilation; reasonably quiet; regular hours.	5
2.	Comfortable conditions; occasional noise or irregular hours; limited exposure to disagreeable work elements.	10
3.	Comfortable conditions; periodic disagreeable noise or scheduled overtime or weekend hours; regular exposure to disagreeable work elements.	15
4.	Regular exposure to uncomfortable conditions; constant noise; continuous exposure to disagreeable work elements.	20

Factor #8

Work Environment (Continued)

Degree	Definition	Points
5.	Constant exposure to uncomfortable conditions; constant exposure to disagreeable work elements requiring periodic relief in order to continue working.	25

FACTOR #9

HAZARDS

Hazards refers to inherent job conditions which potentially endanger the health and safety of the job incumbent, such as radiation, patient behavior, stress situations, moving machinery, etc. Both probability and severity of injury or illness are considered.

This factor is rated on overall exposure, assuming that reasonable care is exercised in observing safety rules and health regulations.

Degree	Definition	Points
1.	Apparent hazards limited to exposure similar to that involved in normal office routine.	5
2.	Exposure to injury limited to minor burns, cuts or bruises, or stress from occasional minor abuse from patients or public on questions of service, billing, care, etc.	10
3.	Regular exposure to burns, cuts, bruises, etc., usually causing major personal discomfort, but not loss of work; or work requiring regular explanations of service, etc., with failure generating abuse from the public.	15

Factor #9

Hazards (Continued)

Degree	Definition	Points
4.	Regular exposure to hazards, radiation or infectious materials, likely to produce injuries or illnesses involving loss of time from work; or work involving extreme misunderstandings or abuse from the public, with little recourse to supportive higher authority.	20
5.	Regular exposure to hazards, radiation or infectious materials likely to result in partial or total disability or possible loss of life.	25

FACTOR #10

PERSONAL DEMANDS

Personal demands refers to the physical demands, such as awkward positions, heavy lifting, etc., and the mental demands, such as concentration, attention, perception, etc.

The degree selected for this factor should relate to the average level of effort, reflecting both the average exertion and the continuity required throughout a day's work.

Degree	Definition	Points
1.	Light, occasional physical effort; normal workplace attention and perception required.	10
2.	Light, regular physical demand, such as constant standing or walking; close attention, such as observation of monitors, etc.	20
3.	Majority of time requires considerable effort, either mental or physical; e.g., constant standing or walking with regular lifting or periods of concentration; continuous concentration on detailed reports, calculations, etc.	30

Factor #10

Personal Demands (Continued)

Degree	Definition	Points
4.	Constant heavy work and difficult work positions, or heavy work mixed with periods of constant attention; or regular stress to meet schedules or deadlines involving complex contracts, etc.	40
5.	Hard physical labor, such as unloading trucks, or constant lifting of patients; job is characterized by exertion and fatigue.	50

IV. GENERIC DESCRIPTIONS AND EVALUATIONS

APPENDIX A

IV. Generic Descriptions and Evaluations

Radiology

Clinical Laboratory

Central Service

Nursing Service

Dietetics

Dietetics (Continued)

Housekeeping

Plant Engineering

Purchasing

Financial Management

Rehabilitation

Technical Services

Laundry

Medical Records

Personnel

JOB DESCRIPTION

Job Title: Chief Radiologic Technologist

Department: Radiology

Primary Function: Plans, organizes, supervises and evaluates department performance in regard to technical services and personnel; responsible for maintenance of quality technical service.

Reports To (Title):

Supervises (Title):

Typical Duties:

Ensures radiologic services are maintained in accordance with established standards of the hospital, state, local, and federal regulations.

Coordinates requests for services and makes work assignments to expedite all aspects of radiologic function.

Schedules, supervises, and evaluates department personnel.

Interviews, selects, and orients new employees.

Conducts in-service training and demonstrates new or difficult procedures to technical staff.

Evaluates and ensures the accuracy and technical quality of X-rays.

Prepares department reports and documentation.

Ensures proper equipment maintenance and usage, and maintains records of maintenance and repair.

Develops and recommends new or modified technical procedures and equipment.

Coordinates departmental purchasing to maintain adequate stock levels, storage and utilization procedures.

Advises supervisor of department status.

Performs general technical duties when work load is heavy.

Job Title: Chief Radiologic Technologist (Continued)

Prerequisites: Graduation from an accredited school of radiologic technology training and registered by the American Registry of Radiologic Technologists (ART).

Working Conditions:

APPROVED:	REVIEWED AND RETAINED:
______________________	______________________
Supervisor	Supervisor
______________________	______________________
Date	Date
______________________	______________________
Department Head	Department Head
______________________	______________________
Date	Date

JOB TITLE: CHIEF RADIOLOGIC TECHNOLOGIST DATE:

	BASIS OF EVALUATION	POINTS
SKILL	FACTOR #1 - MENTAL DEVELOPMENT -- Requires specific knowledge of principles of a specialized field and their applications Benchmark Reference(s):	60
	FACTOR #2 - WORK EXPERIENCE -- Management of an overall function Benchmark Reference(s):	75
	FACTOR #3 - JUDGMENT -- Majority of time spent in decision making regarding personnel and procedures Benchmark Reference(s):	40
RESPONSIBILITY	FACTOR #4 - ERRORS AND LOSSES -- Constant care required to assure compliance with regulations Benchmark Reference(s):	40
	FACTOR #5 - RESOURCE UTILIZATION -- Responsible for effective utilization of department facilities and its' employees, inventory, equipment and planning Benchmark Reference(s):	40
	FACTOR #6 - SYSTEMS AND DATA -- Responsible for all radiology - serious consequences to hospital if not adequate Benchmark Reference(s):	50
	FACTOR #7 - INTERPERSONAL RELATIONSHIPS -- Coordinates radiology activity with other hospital personnel and functions, resolves conflicts Benchmark Reference(s):	60
WORKING CONDITIONS	FACTOR #8 - WORK ENVIRONMENT -- Comfortable conditions Benchmark Reference(s):	10
	FACTOR #9 - HAZARDS -- Regular exposure to radiation Benchmark Reference(s):	20
EFFORT	FACTOR #10 - PERSONAL DEMANDS -- Considerable effort and stress Benchmark Reference(s):	30

TOTAL POINT EVALUATION: 425

JOB DESCRIPTION

Job Title: Radiologic Technologist

Department: Radiology

Primary Function: Sets up and operates X-ray equipment to produce standard and special radiographs of portions of the body for purpose of diagnosis and treatment.

Reports To (Title):

Supervises (Title):

Typical Duties:

Positions and adjusts equipment to proper setting for each examination.

Prepares patient for X-ray and explains procedure.

Assists patient on and off of X-ray table and positions patient using supportive and immobilization equipment as required.

Matches X-ray film to patient report form in preparation for interpretation by radiologist.

Assists radiologist in performing fluoroscopic examinations and x-ray therapy machines.

Prepares and administers chemical mixture to patient under direction of radiologist.

Develops film.

Prepares and maintains adequate records and files.

Maintains equipment in proper working order.

Observes radiation safety standards.

Maintains a clean and orderly work environment.

Secures and returns supplies.

Prerequisites: Graduation from an accredited school of radiologic technology and registered by the American Registry of Radiologic Technologists (ART).

Job Title: Radiologic Technologist (Continued)

Working Conditions:

APPROVED:	REVIEWED AND RETAINED:
Supervisor	Supervisor
Date	Date
Department Head	Department Head
Date	Date

JOB TITLE: RADIOLOGIC TECHNOLOGIST DATE:

	BASIS OF EVALUATION	POINTS
SKILL	FACTOR #1 - MENTAL DEVELOPMENT -- Knowledge of a specialized field required Benchmark Reference(s):	45
	FACTOR #2 - WORK EXPERIENCE -- Must learn work layout and recording procedures Benchmark Reference(s):	30
	FACTOR #3 - JUDGMENT -- Detailed job procedures, decisions within established guidelines Benchmark Reference(s):	30
RESPONSIBILITY	FACTOR #4 - ERRORS AND LOSSES -- Considerable care required in determining radiation levels and observing safety standards Benchmark Reference(s):	30
	FACTOR #5 - RESOURCE UTILIZATION -- Requires care for efficient operation Benchmark Reference(s):	20
	FACTOR #6 - SYSTEMS AND DATA -- Part of radiation team, not critical to functioning of hospital Benchmark Reference(s):	30
	FACTOR #7 - INTERPERSONAL RELATIONSHIPS --Frequent and substantive contact with patients, following standard procedures Benchmark Reference(s):	45
WORKING CONDITIONS	FACTOR #8 - WORK ENVIRONMENT -- Comfortable conditions Benchmark Reference(s):	10
	FACTOR #9 - HAZARDS -- Regular exposure to radiation Benchmark Reference(s):	20
EFFORT	FACTOR #10 - PERSONAL DEMANDS -- Close attention required to assure quality X-ray or radiation results Benchmark Reference(s):	20

TOTAL POINT EVALUATION: 280

JOB DESCRIPTION

Job Title: Chief Laboratory Technologist

Department: Clinical Laboratory

Primary Function: Plans, coordinates and supervises laboratory activities to assure that all laboratory procedures adhere to hospital and governmental guidelines, that testing results are reported on a timely basis and that safety procedures are followed.

Reports To (Title):

Supervises (Title): Interviews and selects new employees, and provides for their orientation.

Plans and recommends for future department resources including personnel, equipment, space, and general budgeting.

Ensures that hospital and state guidelines are adhered to.

Supervises research and development of new procedures and equipment.

Supervises the requisition of equipment and supplies.

Ensures proper retention and maintenance of department records.

Ensures proper maintenance and care of equipment.

Assists section chiefs with their responsibilities.

Ensures that staff members keep abreast of and comply with current regulations imposed on the laboratory by outside regulatory agencies.

Reviews technical procedures manual and updates or revises procedures to improve and expedite services and to comply with current regulations.

Job Title: Chief Laboratory Technologist (Continued)

Typical Duties: Consults with pathologist regarding technical and/or patient care problems.

Schedules, supervises, and evaluates department personnel.

Represents the laboratory in interdepartmental communications and department head staff meetings.

Implements, reviews and evaluates quality control programs to monitor methodology, equipment and human variables and documents results.

Prerequisites: Graduation from an accredited school of Medical Technology and current registration as a Medical Technologist by the Registry Board of the American Society of Clinical Pathologists.

Demonstrates a thorough knowledge of laboratory procedures, policies and related regulations.

Working Conditions:

APPROVED:	REVIEWED AND RETAINED:
Supervisor	Supervisor
Date	Date
Department Head	Department Head
Date	Date

JOB TITLE: CHIEF LABORATORY TECHNOLOGIST DATE:

	BASIS OF EVALUATION	POINTS
SKILL	FACTOR #1 - MENTAL DEVELOPMENT -- Detailed knowledge of laboratory procedures, related regulations and their applications Benchmark Reference(s):	75
	FACTOR #2 - WORK EXPERIENCE -- Must be able to manage all areas of the lab - an overall function Benchmark Reference(s):	75
	FACTOR #3 - JUDGMENT -- Follows professional standards, majority of time spent in decision making and management Benchmark Reference(s):	40
RESPONSIBILITY	FACTOR #4 - ERRORS AND LOSSES -- Constant care required to assure quality laboratory activities Benchmark Reference(s):	40
	FACTOR #5 - RESOURCE UTILIZATION -- Responsible for effective and efficient use of laboratory supplies and equipment Benchmark Reference(s):	40
	FACTOR #6 - SYSTEMS AND DATA -- Responsible for delivery of accurate timely laboratory results where substandard performance could result in serious consequences for the hospital Benchmark Reference(s):	50
	FACTOR #7 - INTERPERSONAL RELATIONSHIPS -- Represents department, serves as liaison, coordinates activities Benchmark Reference(s):	60
WORKING CONDITIONS	FACTOR #8 - WORK ENVIRONMENT -- Comfortable conditions Benchmark Reference(s):	10
	FACTOR #9 - HAZARDS -- Must coordinate service with other departments and resolve complaints Benchmark Reference(s):	15
EFFORT	FACTOR #10 - PERSONAL DEMANDS -- Must keep abreast of all lab activities, new technical developments Benchmark Reference(s):	30

TOTAL POINT EVALUATION: 435

JOB DESCRIPTION

Job Title: Medical Laboratory Technician

Department: Clinical Laboratory

Primary Function: Conducts routine tests in the laboratory used in treatment and diagnosis of disease.

Reports To (Title):

Supervises (Title):

Typical Duties:

Performs a variety of routine laboratory procedures within an area of concentration such as histology, hematology, and blood bank, in accordance with established procedures.

Prepares diagnostic material for interpretation; analyzes blood specimens; cross matches and compatibility-tests blood; issues and prepares blood components; and/or performs other similar procedures.

Draws blood from patients for analysis and testing, and/or obtains other specimens as required.

Organizes specimens to ensure that the patient name and number correlates to requisition.

Obtains orders and reference data.

Keeps detailed records of all tests performed.

Prepares solutions, reagents and stains.

Participates in quality control program.

Cleans and maintains equipment in good condition.

Maintains a clean and orderly work environment.

Prerequisites: Certification as a Medical Technician by the Board of Registry of Medical Technologists of the American Society of Clinical Pathologists.

Job Title: Medical Laboratory Technician (Continued)

Working Conditions:

APPROVED:	REVIEWED AND RETAINED:
______________________ Supervisor	______________________ Supervisor
______________________ Date	______________________ Date
______________________ Department Head	______________________ Department Head
______________________ Date	______________________ Date

JOB TITLE: MEDICAL LABORATORY TECHNICIAN DATE:

	BASIS OF EVALUATION	POINTS
SKILL	FACTOR #1 - MENTAL DEVELOPMENT -- Requires knowledge to perform routine lab tests Benchmark Reference(s):	30
	FACTOR #2 - WORK EXPERIENCE -- Must learn lab policies and procedures Benchmark Reference(s):	30
	FACTOR #3 - JUDGMENT -- Follows standard procedures, some judgment in interpreting test results Benchmark Reference(s):	30
RESPONSIBILITY	FACTOR #4 - ERRORS AND LOSSES -- Constant attention required to assure quality test results Benchmark Reference(s):	40
	FACTOR #5 - RESOURCE UTILIZATION -- Uses equipment and materials which require care for efficient operation Benchmark Reference(s):	20
	FACTOR #6 - SYSTEMS AND DATA -- Part of team processing blood, etc., on a timely basis, so as not to interrupt patient care Benchmark Reference(s):	30
	FACTOR #7 - INTERPERSONAL RELATIONSHIPS -- Daily contact with patients to obtain specimens or draw bloods Benchmark Reference(s):	30
WORKING CONDITIONS	FACTOR #8 - WORK ENVIRONMENT -- Regular exposure to fumes, odors in laboratory Benchmark Reference(s):	15
	FACTOR #9 - HAZARDS -- Exposure to infectious materials; chemicals, heat, flame, etc. Benchmark Reference(s):	20
EFFORT	FACTOR #10 - PERSONAL DEMANDS -- Close attention to perform routine tests, constant standing Benchmark Reference(s):	20

TOTAL POINT EVALUATION: 265

JOB DESCRIPTION

Job Title: Medical Technologist (MTASCP)

Department: Clinical Laboratory

Primary Function: Performs numerous clinical procedures for chemical, microscopic, and/or bacteriologic tests in hematology, serology, parasitology and/or blood banking to obtain data for use in diagnosis and treatment of disease and determines whether results are within established limits.

Reports To (Title):

Supervises (Title):

Typical Duties:

Performs quantitative and qualitative laboratory analyses and ensures accuracy by use of quality control programs.

Sets up and operates department instruments and equipment in prescribed manner.

Observes reactions, changes of color, or formation of precipitates studies slides and maintains accurate record of test results.

Organizes samples to be tested in an efficient and accurate manner.

Reviews and suggests improvements to existing procedures.

Organizes and prepares specimens to be sent to referral labs and acts as liaison if assigned.

Prepares reagents and media, and helps inventory and replenish supplies.

Assists in evaluating and instructing affiliated students.

Obtains laboratory specimens directly from patient, unit, or specified source, using established techniques.

Maintains a clean and orderly work environment.

Job Title: Medical Technologist (MTASCP) (Continued)

Typical Duties: Consults with laboratory supervisor and/or pathologist concerning technical and/or patient care problems.

Maintains appropriate records of test results and work activities.

Prerequisites: Graduation from an accredited school of Medical Technology and current registration as a Medical Technologist by the Registry Board of the American Society of Clinical Pathologists.

Working Conditions:

APPROVED:	REVIEWED AND RETAINED:
Supervisor	Supervisor
Date	Date
Department Head	Department Head
Date	Date

JOB TITLE: MEDICAL TECHNOLOGIST (MTASCP) DATE:

	BASIS OF EVALUATION	POINTS
SKILL	FACTOR #1 - MENTAL DEVELOPMENT--Knowledge of a specialized field required Benchmark Reference(s):	45
	FACTOR #2 - WORK EXPERIENCE -- Proficiency in lab procedures is required to carry out job routines Benchmark Reference(s):	45
	FACTOR #3 - JUDGMENT -- Standard professional procedures and practices followed, some judgment in interpretation of test results Benchmark Reference(s):	30
RESPONSIBILITY	FACTOR #4 - ERRORS AND LOSSES -- Constant care required to preserve specimens and assure tests are properly conducted Benchmark Reference(s):	40
	FACTOR #5 - RESOURCE UTILIZATION -- Uses expensive equipment, directs activities of those assigned to assist Benchmark Reference(s):	30
	FACTOR #6 - SYSTEMS AND DATA -- Performs testing on a timely basis, reports results Benchmark Reference(s):	30
	FACTOR #7 - INTERPERSONAL RELATIONSHIPS -- Takes specimens, works with outpatients Benchmark Reference(s):	30
WORKING CONDITIONS	FACTOR #8 - WORK ENVIRONMENT -- Regular exposure to disagreeable work elements such as fumes, odors and chemical solutions Benchmark Reference(s):	15
	FACTOR #9 - HAZARDS -- Exposure to infectious materials, chemicals, heat, flame, etc. Benchmark Reference(s):	20
EFFORT	FACTOR #10 - PERSONAL DEMANDS -- Continuous concentration in care to perform tests Benchmark Reference(s):	30

TOTAL POINT EVALUATION: 315

JOB DESCRIPTION

Job Title: Laboratory Supervisor (Section)

Department: Clinical Laboratory

Primary Function: Supervises and coordinates activities of employees performing bacteriological, serological, hemotological and related examinations. Assists in testing and performs various special testing procedures as required.

Reports To (Title):

Supervises (Title):

Typical Duties: Supervises and coordinates activities of support personnel to ensure quality technical services.

Ensures procedures are done when scheduled.

Schedules personnel and ensures proper section coverage.

Performs special, sophisicated, technical and/or experimental testing procedures as required.

Monitors validity and accuracy of tests performed by assigned personnel and monitors test records to ensure test results are within accepted quality control ranges.

Assists in the evaluation of new procedures and equipment in department.

Establishes and implements routine instrument and equipment maintenance program.

Participates in the requisition of equipment and supplies.

Assists with routine and nonroutine procedures when needed.

Assists in the maintenance and care of equipment.

Job Title: Laboratory Supervisor (Continued)

Typical Duties:

Ensures that lab sections records are accurate, up-to-date and within hospital policies and procedures.

Keeps abreast of new developments in test methods and procedures.

Assures that assigned personnel adhere to hospital safety policies and procedures.

Participates in in-service education programs and helps instruct affiliated students.

Consults with the medical technologist and/or pathologist in charge of the section regarding technical or patient care problems.

Communicates with patients' physicians concerning abnormal test results.

Prerequisites: Graduation from an accredited school of Medical Technology and current registration as a Medical Technologist by the Registry Board of the American Society of Clinical Pathologists.

Working Conditions:

APPROVED:	REVIEWED AND RETAINED:
Supervisor	Supervisor
Date	Date
Department Head	Department Head
Date	Date

JOB TITLE: LABORATORY SUPERVISOR DATE:

	BASIS OF EVALUATION	POINTS
SKILL	FACTOR #1 - MENTAL DEVELOPMENT -- Must have specific knowledge of all operations performed within a section of the laboratory Benchmark Reference(s):	60
	FACTOR #2 - WORK EXPERIENCE -- Must be able to supervise all activities in a lab section Benchmark Reference(s):	60
	FACTOR #3 - JUDGMENT -- Follows professional standards and hospital procedures Benchmark Reference(s):	30
RESPONSIBILITY	FACTOR #4 - ERRORS AND LOSSES -- Constant care required to assure quality results in lab section Benchmark Reference(s):	40
	FACTOR #5 - RESOURCE UTILIZATION -- Assures efficient use of supplies and equipment in lab section Benchmark Reference(s):	30
	FACTOR #6 - SYSTEMS AND DATA -- Responsible for delivery of timely, accurate laboratory results and feedback for a lab section Benchmark Reference(s):	40
	FACTOR #7 - INTERPERSONAL RELATIONSHIPS -- Supervisory responsibility for a section Benchmark Reference(s):	45
WORKING CONDITIONS	FACTOR #8 - WORK ENVIRONMENT -- Regular exposure to disagreeable work conditions - fumes, odors Benchmark Reference(s):	15
	FACTOR #9 - HAZARDS -- Exposure to infectious materials, chemicals, heat, flames, etc. Benchmark Reference(s):	20
EFFORT	FACTOR #10 - PERSONAL DEMANDS -- Continuous concentration and care to perform tests Benchmark Reference(s):	30

TOTAL POINT EVALUATION: 370

JOB DESCRIPTION

Job Title: Laboratory Aide

Department: Clinical Laboratory

Primary Function: Cleans glassware, instruments, work tables and other laboratory equipment and assists laboratory personnel with routine duties as requested

Reports To (Title):

Supervises (Title):

Typical Duties:

Prepares cleaning solutions as specified and uses them to properly clean glassware and equipment.

Sterilizes glassware and instruments using autoclave.

Examines cleaned equipment to inspect for damage or breakage and discards.

Distributes cleaned items to their proper location in lab.

Participates in the storage and inventory of supplies.

Obtains and distributes supplies on a daily basis.

Maintains proper care of refrigeration units and autoclave.

Runs errands as requested.

Maintains a clean and orderly work environment.

Assists with other related duties as assigned.

Performs simple laboratory tests under close supervision.

Keeps records of specimens held in laboratory.

Prerequisites: None

Job Title: Laboratory Aide (Continued)

Working Conditions:

APPROVED:	REVIEWED AND RETAINED:
Supervisor	Supervisor
Date	Date
Department Head	Department Head
Date	Date

JOB TITLE: LABORATORY AIDE DATE:

	BASIS OF EVALUATION	POINTS
SKILL	FACTOR #1 - MENTAL DEVELOPMENT -- No special knowledge required Benchmark Reference(s):	15
	FACTOR #2 - WORK EXPERIENCE -- Normal indoctrination to lab support procedures Benchmark Reference(s):	15
	FACTOR #3 - JUDGMENT -- Little variation in work routine Benchmark Reference(s):	10
RESPONSIBILITY	FACTOR #4 - ERRORS AND LOSSES -- Work closely supervised Benchmark Reference(s):	10
	FACTOR #5 - RESOURCE UTILIZATION -- Controls or impacts few resources of the hospital Benchmark Reference(s):	10
	FACTOR #6 - SYSTEMS AND DATA -- Member of lab team, duties can be checked and performed by other team members Benchmark Reference(s):	20
	FACTOR #7 - INTERPERSONAL RELATIONSHIPS -- Assist others Benchmark Reference(s):	15
WORKING CONDITIONS	FACTOR #8 - WORK ENVIRONMENT -- Regular exposure to disagreeable elements Benchmark Reference(s):	15
	FACTOR #9 - HAZARDS -- Exposure to infectious materials, chemicals, heat, flame, etc. Benchmark Reference(s):	20
EFFORT	FACTOR #10 - PERSONAL DEMANDS -- Normal work place attention and perception required Benchmark Reference(s):	10

TOTAL POINT EVALUATION: 140

JOB DESCRIPTION

Job Title: Central Service Technician

Department: Central Service

Primary Function: Carries out cleaning, sterilizing and assembly procedures to maintain reusable equipment, instruments and supplies.

Reports To (Title):

Supervises (Title):

Typical Duties:

Cleans, inspects, and maintains surgical instruments and equipment.

Washes and inspects tray wrappers and sheets.

Decontaminates and sterilizes instruments and equipment.

Packages supplies and instrument trays according to designated procedures and labels them.

Operates steam and gas sterilizers as prescribed.

Notifies appropriate personnel of equipment malfunctions.

Redates all sterile articles as prescribed.

Collects, cleans, inspects, sterilizes and returns equipment stored in hospital utility rooms.

Dispenses sterile items and receives dirty items at the respective work stations.

Delivers sterile syringes and trays to nursing units as required.

Maintains appropriate records to assist in the control of central supply inventory.

Obtains needed equipment on an emergency basis from other departments, other hospitals, or through the purchasing department.

Job Title: Central Service Technician (Continued)

Prerequisites: Successful completion of on-the-job training program.

Working Conditions:

APPROVED:	REVIEWED AND RETAINED:
______________________	______________________
Supervisor	Supervisor
______________________	______________________
Date	Date
______________________	______________________
Department Head	Department Head
______________________	______________________
Date	Date

JOB TITLE: CENTRAL SERVICE TECHNICIAN DATE:

	BASIS OF EVALUATION	POINTS
SKILL	FACTOR #1 - MENTAL DEVELOPMENT -- No specialized knowledge required Benchmark Reference(s):	15
	FACTOR #2 - WORK EXPERIENCE -- Completion of on-the-job training program Benchmark Reference(s):	30
	FACTOR #3 - JUDGMENT -- Routines prescribed Benchmark Reference(s):	10
RESPONSIBILITY	FACTOR #4 - ERRORS AND LOSSES -- Normal care required to assure machines functioning properly, items are processed and assembled correctly. Benchmark Reference(s):	20
	FACTOR #5 - RESOURCE UTILIZATION -- Utilize a variety of expensive equipment and instruments and supplies Benchmark Reference(s):	20
	FACTOR #6 - SYSTEMS AND DATA -- Responsible for maintaining flow of sterilized and cleaned items available for reuse. Benchmark Reference(s):	20
	FACTOR #7 - INTERPERSONAL RELATIONSHIPS -- Few contacts outside unit Benchmark Reference(s):	15
WORKING CONDITIONS	FACTOR #8 - WORK ENVIRONMENT -- Regular exposure to disagreeable elements Benchmark Reference(s):	15
	FACTOR #9 - HAZARDS -- Frequent possibility of burns, cuts, regular exposure to infectious materials Benchmark Reference(s):	20
EFFORT	FACTOR #10 - PERSONAL DEMANDS -- Continuous standing, stooping and bending Benchmark Reference(s):	30

TOTAL POINT EVALUATION: 195

JOB DESCRIPTION

Job Title:	Staff Nurse
Department:	Nursing Service
Primary Function:	Renders and ensures professional nursing care to patients as directed by the medical staff and in accordance with the hospital's objectives and policies.
Reports To (Title):	
Supervises (Title):	
Typical Duties:	Formulates and implements a nursing care plan for assigned patients and reviews and updates them as required.

Assists in planning, supervising and instructing LPNs, nursing assistants and ancillary personnel and ensures proper and complete discharge of physicians' orders on patient care and treatment.

Administers specific medications at designated times and in designated manner.

Ensures accurate medication is administered, in correct form and dosage to proper patient as ordered by physician.

Charts medication, dosage and time given and indicates if not administered.

Observes patients, reports any reaction to medication or treatments.

Administers IVs, oversees their proper function and prepares IV medication.

Charts nursing observations and ensures record is complete with all actions and test results recorded.

Makes rounds to assess patients' status, assists with responding to call lights and with patient care.

Checks medicine and drug stocks to ensure adequate supplies.

Job Title: Staff Nurse (Continued)

Typical Duties: Prepares equipment and assists physicians with treatment procedures.

Administers emergency procedures when required.

Participates in in-service education programs.

Explains procedures and treatments to patient to allay fears and gain cooperation.

Prerequisites: Graduate of an accredited school of Nursing and a current license to practice Nursing from the State Board of Nursing.

Working Conditions:

APPROVED:	REVIEWED AND RETAINED:
Supervisor	Supervisor
Date	Date
Department Head	Department Head
Date	Date

JOB TITLE: STAFF NURSE DATE:

	BASIS OF EVALUATION	POINTS
SKILL	FACTOR #1 - MENTAL DEVELOPMENT -- Specific knowledge of nursing principles and patient care procedures. 2 years specialized training and state license Benchmark Reference(s):	45
	FACTOR #2 - WORK EXPERIENCE -- Proficiency in lower level nursing activities, such as LPN, Nursing Assistant responsibilities required Benchmark Reference(s):	45
	FACTOR #3 - JUDGMENT -- Follows professional and hospital standard practice, solves specific problems, (e.g. emergencies) from time to time Benchmark Reference(s):	30
RESPONSIBILITY	FACTOR #4 - ERRORS AND LOSSES -- Requires constant care to properly administer drugs and patient care Benchmark Reference(s):	40
	FACTOR #5 - RESOURCE UTILIZATION -- Directs group of LPN's, nursing assistants, monitors inventory levels Benchmark Reference(s):	30
	FACTOR #6 - SYSTEMS AND DATA -- Responsible for system of patient care for an assigned group of patients Benchmark Reference(s):	40
	FACTOR #7 - INTERPERSONAL RELATIONSHIPS -- Frequent contacts with patients, families and other departments of a variable nature Benchmark Reference(s):	45
WORKING CONDITIONS	FACTOR #8 - WORK ENVIRONMENT -- Scheduled weekend hours, attends to patient bodily needs Benchmark Reference(s):	15
	FACTOR #9 - HAZARDS -- Some exposure to infectious materials, sharp instruments Benchmark Reference(s):	15
EFFORT	FACTOR #10 - PERSONAL DEMANDS -- Regular physical and mental effort Benchmark Reference(s):	20

TOTAL POINT EVALUATION: 325

JOB DESCRIPTION

Job Title: Instructor, Staff Development

Department: Nursing Service

Primary Function: Plans, develops, and conducts in-service education and orientation programs for all hospital nursing service personnel and develops programs for on-going staff development.

Reports To (Title):

Supervises (Title):

Typical Duties:

Conducts orientation program for all new Nursing Service employees to ensure their knowledge of hospital policy and procedure.

Assists in planning and conducting continuing educational programs for all nursing service personnel to update and maintain high standards of nursing care.

Attends seminars, workshops and conferences to remain up-to-date with the latest skills, procedures and techniques to assure continuous professional growth.

Serves as a member of various committees as representative of nursing department and incorporates changes into teaching programs and policy and procedure manuals.

Prepares reports on external continuing education programs.

Evaluates the effectiveness of staff development programs and prepares evaluations of nursing staff in collaboration with nursing supervision.

Instructs hospital employees and physicians as needed in all types of patient therapies such as: respirator care, CPR, various punctures, biopsies, and other diagnostic or treatment procedures.

Acts as facilitator and resource person in clinical teaching and committee work. Provides informational material to meet needs of unit staff and to find solutions to patient care problems.

Job Title: Instructor, Staff Development (Continued)

Prerequisites: Graduation from an accredited school of Nursing and a current license from the State Board of Nursing.

Working Conditions:

APPROVED:	REVIEWED AND RETAINED:
Supervisor	Supervisor
Date	Date
Department Head	Department Head
Date	Date

JOB TITLE: INSTRUCTOR - STAFF DEVELOPMENT DATE:

	BASIS OF EVALUATION	POINTS
SKILL	FACTOR #1 - MENTAL DEVELOPMENT -- Knowledge of principles of nursing and ability to teach required Benchmark Reference(s):	60
	FACTOR #2 - WORK EXPERIENCE -- Must be experienced in various nursing specialities to provide orientation and in-service instruction Benchmark Reference(s):	60
	FACTOR #3 - JUDGMENT -- General policies established, judgment in designing and implementing programs required Benchmark Reference(s):	40
RESPONSIBILITY	FACTOR #4 - ERRORS AND LOSSES -- Loosely supervised; must be very careful to explain procedures properly Benchmark Reference(s):	40
	FACTOR #5 - RESOURCE UTILIZATION -- Responsibility to use training time effectively and to assure sufficient knowledge in new employees Benchmark Reference(s):	30
	FACTOR #6 - SYSTEMS AND DATA -- Responsible for in-house training and education process Benchmark Reference(s):	40
	FACTOR #7 - INTERPERSONAL RELATIONSHIPS -- Exposed to nearly all nursing service personnel as teacher Benchmark Reference(s):	75
WORKING CONDITIONS	FACTOR #8 - WORK ENVIRONMENT -- Occasional clinical teaching, irregular hours Benchmark Reference(s):	10
	FACTOR #9 - HAZARDS -- Instructs in use of nursing equipment Benchmark Reference(s):	10
EFFORT	FACTOR #10 - PERSONAL DEMANDS -- Some standing, walking, must respond to questions Benchmark Reference(s):	20

TOTAL POINT EVALUATION: 385

JOB DESCRIPTION

Job Title: Nursing Assistant

Department: Nursing Service

Primary Function: Provides direct patient care encompassing admission process, physical hygiene and treatment intervention within limits of authority.

Reports To (Title):

Supervises (Title):

Typical Duties:

Bathes patients and otherwise assists with personal hygiene to maximize their comfort, including bed baths, tub baths and showers, oral hygiene, care of hair, fingernails, etc.

Serves and collects food trays, prepares patients for meals, feeds patients as required, and provides nourishments and fresh water when indicated.

Monitors patients, recognizing and reporting adverse symptoms and reactions.

Checks blood pressure, temperature, respiration, intake and output, weight, and records results.

Changes bed linen of both occupied and unoccupied beds and tidies patients' rooms.

Responds to call lights, determines patients' needs and reports unusual changes in status.

Assists in moving and lifting of patients both in and out of bed by manual and mechanical means, and walks patients for exercise.

Applies hot water bottle, compresses, alcohol sponge and changes some dressings.

Applies binders and bandages when ordered by physician and prevents and treats bedsores.

Administers cleansing enema, Harris flush, and retention enema when ordered by physician.

Job Title: Nursing Assistant (Continued)

Typical Duties: Collects stools, urine and sputum specimens as ordered by physician and tests urine for sugar and acetone.

Assists in admission, discharge, and transfer of patients.

Participates in in-service programs.

Runs errands and performs other related duties as required.

Prerequisites: Successful completion of on-the-job training program.

Working Conditions:

APPROVED:

____
Supervisor

____
Date

____
Department Head

____
Date

REVIEWED AND RETAINED:

____
Supervisor

____
Date

____
Department Head

____
Date

JOB TITLE: NURSING ASSISTANT DATE:

	BASIS OF EVALUATION	POINTS
SKILL	FACTOR #1 - MENTAL DEVELOPMENT -- Ability to read and write required, no specialized knowledge necessary Benchmark Reference(s):	15
	FACTOR #2 - WORK EXPERIENCE -- Completion of formal on-the-job training to learn routines and procedures Benchmark Reference(s):	30
	FACTOR #3 - JUDGMENT -- Prescribed routines, some judgment in patient handling Benchmark Reference(s):	20
RESPONSIBILITY	FACTOR #4 - ERRORS AND LOSSES -- Normal care necessary, close review of work by others Benchmark Reference(s):	20
	FACTOR #5 - RESOURCE UTILIZATION -- Uses materials and supplies as directed Benchmark Reference(s):	10
	FACTOR #6 - SYSTEMS AND DATA -- Works as part of nursing team Benchmark Reference(s):	20
	FACTOR #7 - INTERPERSONAL RELATIONSHIPS -- Routine contacts with patients Benchmark Reference(s):	15
WORKING CONDITIONS	FACTOR #8 - WORK ENVIRONMENT -- Regular exposure to disagreeable elements Benchmark Reference(s):	15
	FACTOR #9 - HAZARDS -- Exposure to infectious materials Benchmark Reference(s):	15
EFFORT	FACTOR #10 - PERSONAL DEMANDS -- Patient lifting Benchmark Reference(s):	30

TOTAL POINT EVALUATION: 190

JOB DESCRIPTION

Job Title: Nursing Supervisor

Department: Nursing Service

Primary Function: Supervises, coordinates and evaluates activities of nursing personnel to ensure quality patient care in accordance with hospital policy within the specific locations of the hospital and nursing units to which they are assigned.

Reports To (Title):

Supervises (Title):

Typical Duties:

Supervises carrying out responsibilities in the management of nursing care.

Determines staffing needs of hospital and provides for staffing of all nursing units.

Inspects and evaluates unit areas to assure the delivery of safe, efficient, and effective patient care.

Coordinates service to patient with other patient care units and related departments.

Consults on the interpretation and implementation of hospital policies and procedures.

Assists in evaluating nursing service performance; selecting new employees; ensuring proper coverage and scheduling of personnel.

Assists in the resolution of problems, complaints and emergencies.

Supervises maintenance of personnel and nursing records.

Supports, works collaboratively and participates in guidance and educational programs.

Participates in activities to further professional growth, knowledge, and improving nursing care.

Assists in formulating unit budget.

Job Title: Nursing Supervisor (Continued)

Prerequisites:

Working Conditions:

APPROVED:	REVIEWED AND RETAINED:
Supervisor	Supervisor
Date	Date
Department Head	Department Head
Date	Date

JOB TITLE: NURSING SUPERVISOR DATE:

	BASIS OF EVALUATION	POINTS
SKILL	FACTOR #1 - MENTAL DEVELOPMENT -- Requires knowledge of principles of nursing field and their applications Benchmark Reference(s):	60
SKILL	FACTOR #2 - WORK EXPERIENCE -- Proficiency in all nursing care, supervises large number of people engaged in various activities Benchmark Reference(s):	60
SKILL	FACTOR #3 - JUDGMENT -- Deals with emergencies, provides technical assistance, responds to any irregularity in hospital procedures Benchmark Reference(s):	40
RESPONSIBILITY	FACTOR #4 - ERRORS AND LOSSES -- Highest ranking personnel in-house on shift Benchmark Reference(s):	50
RESPONSIBILITY	FACTOR #5 - RESOURCE UTILIZATION -- Responsible for efficient utilization of resources during shift Benchmark Reference(s):	50
RESPONSIBILITY	FACTOR #6 - SYSTEMS AND DATA -- Responsible for health care delivery for entire shift Benchmark Reference(s):	50
RESPONSIBILITY	FACTOR #7 - INTERPERSONAL RELATIONSHIPS -- Deals with any irregularities or problems not able to be resolved by others in shift Benchmark Reference(s):	60
WORKING CONDITIONS	FACTOR #8 - WORK ENVIRONMENT -- Comfortable conditions Benchmark Reference(s):	10
WORKING CONDITIONS	FACTOR #9 - HAZARDS -- Stress element of position of authority Benchmark Reference(s):	15
EFFORT	FACTOR #10 - PERSONAL DEMANDS -- Continuous concentration Benchmark Reference(s):	30

TOTAL POINT EVALUATION: 425

JOB DESCRIPTION

Job Title: Unit Clerk/Unit Secretary

Department: Nursing Service

Primary Function: Performs routine clerical duties and receptionist functions for hospital nursing unit.

Reports To (Title):

Supervises (Title):

Typical Duties:

Transcribes doctor's orders from charts and records information and test results into computer termimal.

Orders nourishment and supplies for the unit.

Prepares and maintains a file of requisitions and schedules pertinent to the unit.

Answers the phone, takes messages, and dispatches messages both inside and outside the hospital. Establishes good public and hospital relationships.

Requests and schedules special studies and consultations at physicians' request.

Records vital signs, sugar and acetone, intake and output, and test results on patients' charts under the direction of a staff nurse.

Runs errands, obtains X-rays from radiology department, picks up medications and supplies, delivers specimens, and other errands as needed.

Responds to patients' intercoms and helps answer call lights.

Delivers patients' mail, flowers, and gifts promptly and courtesously.

Assists with proper recordkeeping and processing of patients regarding admission, identification, transfer and discharge.

Job Title: Unit Clerk/Unit Secretary (Continued)

Typical Duties: Maintains patient charts in appropriate order, establishing new charts, making notations, transcribing orders and keeping them up-to-date as required.

Participates in in-service education programs.

Performs other related duties as requested.

Prerequisites: Demonstrates a good knowledge of medical terminology. Successful completion of on-the-job training program.

Working Conditions

APPROVED:	REVIEWED AND RETAINED:
Supervisor	Supervisor
Date	Date
Department Head	Department Head
Date	Date

JOB TITLE: UNIT CLERK/UNIT SECRETARY DATE:

	BASIS OF EVALUATION	POINTS
SKILL	FACTOR #1 - MENTAL DEVELOPMENT -- Knowledge of medical terminology required, read and transcribe charts Benchmark Reference(s):	30
	FACTOR #2 - WORK EXPERIENCE -- Completion of formal on-the-job training program required Benchmark Reference(s):	30
	FACTOR #3 - JUDGMENT -- Established hospital procedures must be adhered to Benchmark Reference(s):	20
RESPONSIBILITY	FACTOR #4 - ERRORS AND LOSSES -- Must take normal care in transcription and ordering of supplies, work is reviewed Benchmark Reference(s):	20
	FACTOR #5 - RESOURCE UTILIZATION -- Keeps inventory records Benchmark Reference(s):	20
	FACTOR #6 - SYSTEMS AND DATA -- Provides necessary clerical support to keep nursing unit, billing systems, etc., functioning Benchmark Reference(s):	30
	FACTOR #7 - INTERPERSONAL RELATIONSHIPS -- Regular contacts with other departments, acts as unit receptionist Benchmark Reference(s):	30
WORKING CONDITIONS	FACTOR #8 - WORK ENVIRONMENT -- Irregular hours, comfortable conditions Benchmark Reference(s):	10
	FACTOR #9 - HAZARDS -- Occasional minor abuse from patients, and staff Benchmark Reference(s):	10
EFFORT	FACTOR #10 - PERSONAL DEMANDS -- Must pay close attention when transcribing, ordering supplies Benchmark Reference(s):	20

TOTAL POINT EVALUATION: 220

JOB DESCRIPTION

Job Title: Infection Control Nurse

Department: Nursing Service

Primary Function: Detects, investigates, and reports for managerial action nosocomial infections within the hospital; coordinates and implements infection control procedures; and educates employees in regard to infection prevention and control.

Reports To (Title):

Supervises (Title):

Typical Duties:

Detects and records nosocomial infections on a systematic and current basis and initiates investigation of source.

Advises employees about hospital infection policy and disposition of patients admitted with infection.

Analyzes nosocomial infections with the help of epidemiologist and prepares monthly report for infection control committee.

Assists in in-service training program related to infection prevention and control.

Reports to Health Department all "reportable diseases."

Reviews environmental cleanliness and develops and implements improved infection control methods.

Performs related activities as directed.

Prerequisites: Graduation from an accredited school of Nursing and a current license from the State Board of Nursing.

Working Conditions:

Job Title: Infection Control Nurse (Continued)

APPROVED:	REVIEWED AND RETAINED:
Supervisor	Supervisor
Date	Date
Department Head	Department Head
Date	Date

JOB TITLE: INFECTION CONTROL NURSE DATE:

	BASIS OF EVALUATION	POINTS
SKILL	FACTOR #1 - MENTAL DEVELOPMENT -- Must apply specialized infection control knowledge to all areas of hospital Benchmark Reference(s):	60
SKILL	FACTOR #2 - WORK EXPERIENCE -- Must be proficient in hospital policies and procedures regarding infection control Benchmark Reference(s):	45
SKILL	FACTOR #3 - JUDGMENT -- Administers infection control program within established guidelines Benchmark Reference(s):	30
RESPONSIBILITY	FACTOR #4 - ERRORS AND LOSSES -- Little supervision, constant vigilance required to assure hospital free of infection Benchmark Reference(s):	40
RESPONSIBILITY	FACTOR #5 - RESOURCE UTILIZATION -- Is responsible for the effective utilization of infection control materials Benchmark Reference(s):	30
RESPONSIBILITY	FACTOR #6 SYSTEMS AND DATA -- Administers the infection control program Benchmark Reference(s):	40
RESPONSIBILITY	FACTOR #7 - INTERPERSONAL RELATIONSHIPS -- Interact with nearly all hospital departments, public health agencies Benchmark Reference(s):	45
WORKING CONDITIONS	FACTOR #8 - WORK ENVIRONMENT -- Relatively comfortable conditions, some irregular hours Benchmark Reference(s):	10
WORKING CONDITIONS	FACTOR #9 - HAZARDS -- Some exposures to infectious materials Benchmark Reference(s):	10
EFFORT	FACTOR #10 - PERSONAL DEMANDS -- Regular physical and mental demands Benchmark Reference(s):	20
	TOTAL POINT EVALUATION:	330

JOB DESCRIPTION

Job Title: Licensed Practical Nurse

Department: Nursing Service

Primary Function: Performs assigned nursing procedures for the comfort and well-being of patients.

Reports To (Title):

Supervises (Title):

Typical Duties:

Administers specific medications at designated times and in designated manner.

Ensures accurate medication is administered in correct form and dosage to proper patient as ordered by physician.

Maintains records of nursing care, dose and time of medication administered, and indicates if not administered and reason.

Checks medicines and drug stock to ensure adequate supply and reorders when necessary.

Checks IVs to make certain they are on schedule, running at correct rate of speed and regulates if necessary.

Performs routine nursing care activities such as taking blood pressures, temperatures, baths and hygiene care, passing and removal of trays, changing of linen, and otherwise assists in the care for the physical needs of the patient.

Takes vital signs, observes, monitors and checks for changes in patients' condition.

Answers call lights and assists patients.

Administers treatments, irrigations, enemas, catheters and suctions; changes dressings, applies compresses, and ambulates patients.

Assists with charting of nursing observations, treatments and procedures and transcribes orders when requested.

Monitors patients, recognizing and reporting adverse symptoms or patient reactions.

Job Title: Licensed Practical Nurse (Continued)

Typical Duties:

Sets up trays for procedures and assists physicians with treatments and dressings as requested.

Performs preoperative procedures for surgery or tests, and fills out preop checklist.

Checks emergency cart each shift and replenishes if necessary.

Assists patients in admission, transfer, and discharge procedures.

Assists in emergency procedures such as CPR.

Participates in in-service education programs.

Performs other related duties as requested.

Prerequisites: Graduate of an accredited vocational program for Practical Nursing; completion state required Pharmacology course; and license to practice Licensed Practical Nursing and administer medication from the State Board of Nursing.

Working Conditions:

APPROVED:	REVIEWED AND RETAINED:
______________________ Supervisor	______________________ Supervisor
______________________ Date	______________________ Date
______________________ Department Head	______________________ Department Head
______________________ Date	______________________ Date

JOB TITLE: LPN DATE:

	BASIS OF EVALUATION	POINTS
SKILL	<u>FACTOR #1 - MENTAL DEVELOPMENT</u> -- General knowledge of the basics of nursing Benchmark Reference(s):	30
	<u>FACTOR #2 - WORK EXPERIENCE</u> -- Requires knowledge of hospital policy, procedures and routines Benchmark Reference(s):	30
	<u>FACTOR #3 - JUDGMENT</u> -- Follows prescribed procedures, notifies staff nurse of irregularities Benchmark Reference(s):	20
RESPONSIBILITY	<u>FACTOR #4 - ERRORS AND LOSSES</u> -- Administers medication Benchmark Reference(s):	30
	<u>FACTOR #5 - RESOURCE UTILIZATION</u> -- Uses various nursing supplies Benchmark Reference(s):	20
	<u>FACTOR #6 - SYSTEMS AND DATA</u> -- Shares responsibility as part of nursing team Benchmark Reference(s):	30
	<u>FACTOR #7 - INTERPERSONAL RELATIONSHIPS</u> -- Routine contacts with patients, families, personnel, other departments Benchmark Reference(s):	30
WORKING CONDITIONS	<u>FACTOR #8 - WORK ENVIRONMENT</u> -- Weekend hours - limited exposure to disagreeable elements Benchmark Reference(s):	15
	<u>FACTOR #9 - HAZARDS</u> -- Some exposure to infectious materials and sharp instruments Benchmark Reference(s):	15
EFFORT	<u>FACTOR #10 - PERSONAL DEMANDS</u> -- Patient lifting Benchmark Reference(s):	30

TOTAL POINT EVALUATION: 250

JOB DESCRIPTION

Job Title:	Department Secretary
Department:	Nursing Service
Primary Function:	Performs a variety of secretarial services for the Department of Nursing Service, performs routine clerical functions and implements office procedures for nursing service administration.
Reports To (Title):	
Supervises (Title):	
Typical Duties:	Types correspondence and memos for nursing administration and maintains files. Maintains nursing service personnel salary records. Coordinates arrangements for seminars, workshops, conferences, and classes for nursing service personnel outside of the hospital; and coordinates arrangements for in-service education programs. Maintains and types updates of nursing policy and procedures, job description manuals, minutes of nursing service department meetings, and other reports as requested. Answers phones, responds to routine inquiries, and dispatches messages and information. Interprets and implements policies and procedures as set down by nursing service administration. Assumes duties of other clerical personnel in their absence or when requested. Performs other clerical and adminstrative duties as requested. Demonstrates ability to type 40 wpm.

Job Title: Department Secretary

Working Conditions:

APPROVED:	REVIEWED AND RETAINED:
______________________	______________________
Supervisor	Supervisor
______________________	______________________
Date	Date
______________________	______________________
Department Head	Department Head
______________________	______________________
Date	Date

JOB TITLE: DEPARTMENT SECRETARY DATE:

	BASIS OF EVALUATION	POINTS
SKILL	FACTOR #1 - MENTAL DEVELOPMENT -- Must know medical terminology, nursing policies and procedures, and be proficient in secretarial skills Benchmark Reference(s):	45
	FACTOR #2 - WORK EXPERIENCE -- Proficient in secretarial skills; on-the-job training in hospital nursing policies and procedures required Benchmark Reference(s):	45
	FACTOR #3 - JUDGMENT -- Must follow-up frequently, exercise occasional judgment following business practices Benchmark Reference(s):	30
RESPONSIBILITY	FACTOR #4 - ERRORS AND LOSSES -- Normal care required, under direct supervision Benchmark Reference(s):	20
	FACTOR #5 - RESOURCE UTILIZATION -- Uses office machines, compiles statistical reports Benchmark Reference(s):	20
	FACTOR #6 - SYSTEMS AND DATA -- Handles confidential information regularly, provides clerical support to nursing administrative systems Benchmark Reference(s):	30
	FACTOR #7 - INTERPERSONAL RELATIONSHIPS -- Has frequent phone contacts, arranges seminars, etc. Benchmark Reference(s):	30
WORKING CONDITIONS	FACTOR #8 - WORK ENVIRONMENT -- Pleasant work environment Benchmark Reference(s):	5
	FACTOR #9 - HAZARDS -- Normal office environment Benchmark Reference(s):	5
EFFORT	FACTOR #10 - PERSONAL DEMANDS -- Close attention for proofing and recordkeeping Benchmark Reference(s):	20

TOTAL POINT EVALUATION: 250

JOB DESCRIPTION

Job Title: Head Nurse

Department: Nursing Service

Primary Function: Directs and supervises activities associated with nursing unit and orients and instructs newly employed nurses on hospital policy and procedures regarding patient care.

Reports To (Title):

Supervises (Title):

Typical Duties:

Plans, organizes, directs, and coordinates facilities; evaluates all nursing services to ensure total patient care in accordance with physicians' orders.

Supervises, evaluates, and assists with patient care activities.

Makes rounds to check on condition of patients and ensure proper implementation of nursing care.

Provides assistance, instruction and guidance to newly employed nurses and evaluates their progress.

Directs preparation and maintenance of patient records.

Records nursing observations of patient care.

Evaluates individual work performance and offers guidance when needed.

Identifies problems and assists in their solution.

Communicates with physicians regarding patient care requirements.

Assists in budget planning and operates unit within budget.

Job Title: Head Nurse (Continued)

Prerequisites: Graduation from an accredited school of Nursing and a current license to practice Nursing from the State Board of Nursing.

Working Conditions:

APPROVED:	REVIEWED AND RETAINED:
______________________	______________________
Supervisor	Supervisor
______________________	______________________
Date	Date
______________________	______________________
Department Head	Department Head
______________________	______________________
Date	Date

JOB TITLE: HEAD NURSE DATE:

	BASIS OF EVALUATION	POINTS
SKILL	<u>FACTOR #1 - MENTAL DEVELOPMENT</u> -- Requires ability to train and knowledge of nursing principles and their application Benchmark Reference(s):	60
	<u>FACTOR #2 - WORK EXPERIENCE</u> -- Must supervise and train various levels of nursing service personnel Benchmark Reference(s):	60
	<u>FACTOR #3 - JUDGMENT</u> -- Time spent supervising unit, solving personnel and patient care related problems Benchmark Reference(s):	40
RESPONSIBILITY	<u>FACTOR #4 - ERRORS AND LOSSES</u> -- Requires constant care to avoid errors and for effective, efficient management of the nursing unit Benchmark Reference(s):	40
	<u>FACTOR #5 - RESOURCE UTILIZATION</u> -- Responsible for effective utilization of personnel and equipment on the unit Benchmark Reference(s):	40
	<u>FACTOR #6 - SYSTEMS AND DATA</u> -- Responsible for health care delivery system of an entire unit Benchmark Reference(s):	40
	<u>FACTOR #7 - INTERPERSONAL RELATIONSHIPS</u> -- 24 hour accountability, deals with doctors, patients, visitors, and other departments in difficult or complex situations Benchmark Reference(s):	60
WORKING CONDITIONS	<u>FACTOR #8 - WORK ENVIRONMENT</u> -- Scheduled weekend hours, 24 hour accountability Benchmark Reference(s):	15
	<u>FACTOR #9 - HAZARDS</u> -- Stress in problem solving Benchmark Reference(s):	15
EFFORT	<u>FACTOR #10 - PERSONAL DEMANDS</u> -- Considerable physical and mental effort Benchmark Reference(s):	30

TOTAL POINT EVALUATION: 400

JOB DESCRIPTION

Job Title: Assistant Director, Nursing Service

Department: Nursing Service

Primary Function: Assists in organizing and administering the department and assumes responsibilities assigned on the day, evening or night shift to maintain around-the-clock nursing care.

Reports to (Title):

Supervises (Title):

Typical Duties: Directs and supervises professional nursing and auxiliary personnel in rendering patient care activities.

Assists in the interviewing, selection and evaluation of staff personnel.

Promotes harmonious intradepartmental relationships, and maintains good rapport between physicians, personnel, patients and their families.

Plans and conducts meetings and discussions with nursing administration and staff to encourage participation in formulating departmental policies, promote initiative, solve problems and to interpret new regulations and procedures.

Assists in planning for new and effective utilization of staff time, abilities, and facilities to attain service and educational objectives.

Maintains an effective system of nursing records and reports.

Assists in the review and evaluation of budget requests, and economical use of equipment and supplies.

Participates and initiates, when necessary, studies and research to assess nursing administrative practices and nursing care.

Job Title: Assistant Director, Nursing Service (Continued)

Typical Duties: Participates in activities to further professional growth and knowledge.

Evaluates and recommends selection of supplies, equipment, and nursing procedures for improved patient care.

Prerequisites: Graduation from an accredited school of Nursing and a current license to practice Nursing from the State Board of Nursing.

Demonstrates a thorough knowledge of hospital nursing policies and procedures.

Working Conditions:

APPROVED:	REVIEWED AND RETAINED:
Supervisor	Supervisor
Date	Date
Department Head	Department Head
Date	Date

JOB TITLE: ASSISTANT DIRECTOR, NURSING SERVICE DATE:

	BASIS OF EVALUATION	POINTS
SKILL	FACTOR #1 - MENTAL DEVELOPMENT -- Knowledge of nursing principles and their application is required Benchmark Reference(s):	60
	FACTOR #2 - WORK EXPERIENCE -- Management of the overall nursing function Benchmark Reference(s):	75
	FACTOR #3 - JUDGMENT -- Generally follows professional and hospital's standard practice, but majority of time is spent in administrative decision making Benchmark Reference(s):	40
RESPONSIBILITY	FACTOR #4 - ERRORS AND LOSSES -- Variety of job functions and job routines. Requires constant care-giving, considerable authority Benchmark Reference(s):	40
	FACTOR #5 - RESOURCE UTILIZATION -- Significant budgetary and personnel utilization responsibility Benchmark Reference(s):	50
	FACTOR #6 - SYSTEMS AND DATA -- Responsible for a system of patient care that if not adequate, could cause a problem for the entire hospital Benchmark Reference(s):	50
	FACTOR #7 - INTERPERSONAL RELATIONSHIPS -- Managerial responsibility for nursing Benchmark Reference(s):	75
WORKING CONDITIONS	FACTOR #8 - WORK ENVIRONMENT -- Comfortable conditions. Irregular hours and limited exposure to disagreeable work elements Benchmark Reference(s):	10
	FACTOR #9 - HAZARDS -- Regular stress involved with responsibilities Benchmark Reference(s):	15
EFFORT	FACTOR #10 - PERSONAL DEMANDS -- Majority of time requires mental attention, perception, and concentration to perform a wide variety of job functions Benchmark Reference(s):	30

TOTAL POINT EVALUATION: 445

JOB DESCRIPTION

Job Title: Dietary Tray Handler

Department: Dietetic

Primary Function: Assembles trays for patient meals per menu specifications and delivers trays to correct patient on nursing floors.

Reports To (Title):

Supervises (Title):

Typical Duties:

Works on tray assembly line, and loads completed trays onto food carts.

Serves trays from food carts which have been transported to nursing units.

Delivers menus for the next day to patients.

Unloads dirty trays from food carts following each meal.

Washes food carts after each meal.

Cleans silverware and wraps settings in napkins.

Prepares items for assembly line and sets up work station.

Prepares and transports late trays and nourishments to patient rooms.

Performs other duties as assigned.

Prerequisites: None

Working Conditions:

Job Title: Dietary Tray Handler

APPROVED:

____
Supervisor

____
Date

____
Department Head

____
Date

REVIEWED AND RETAINED:

____
Supervisor

____
Date

____
Department Head

____
Date

JOB TITLE: DIETARY TRAY HANDLER DATE:

	BASIS OF EVALUATION	POINTS
SKILL	FACTOR #1 - MENTAL DEVELOPMENT -- No specialized knowledge required Benchmark Reference(s):	15
	FACTOR #2 - WORK EXPERIENCE -- Normal indoctrination to procedures required Benchmark Reference(s):	15
	FACTOR #3 - JUDGMENT -- Little judgment required Benchmark Reference(s):	10
RESPONSIBILITY	FACTOR #4 - ERRORS AND LOSSES -- Must serve food neatly and efficiently Benchmark Reference(s):	20
	FACTOR #5 - RESOURCE UTILIZATION -- Must not be wasteful of food Benchmark Reference(s):	10
	FACTOR #6 - SYSTEMS AND DATA -- Must function as part of team and keep trayline moving Benchmark Reference(s):	20
	FACTOR #7 - INTERPERSONAL RELATIONSHIPS -- Little or no contact with patients Benchmark Reference(s):	15
WORKING CONDITIONS	FACTOR #8 - WORK ENVIRONMENT -- Regular exposure to disagreeable work elements Benchmark Reference(s):	15
	FACTOR #9 - HAZARDS -- Regular exposure to burns, hazards Benchmark Reference(s):	15
EFFORT	FACTOR #10 - PERSONAL DEMANDS -- Constant standing, some lifting Benchmark Reference(s):	20

TOTAL POINT EVALUATION: 155

JOB DESCRIPTION

Job Title: First Cook

Department: Dietetic

Primary Function: Prepares and cooks food for the hospital patients, staff and/or visitors and supervises and coordinates activities of kitchen workers.

Reports To (Title):

Supervises (Title):

Typical Duties:

Assists with preparation of monthly menus.

Reviews menus to determine type and quantity of meats, vegetables, soup, salad, and desserts to be prepared.

Prepares or oversees the washing, trimming, and cooking of food items.

Measures and mixes ingredients according to recipes using a variety of kitchen utensils and equipment.

Ensures sanitary conditions and maintains a clean working area.

Inspects food to ensure freshness of ingredients.

Follows safety procedures regarding the handling of knives, slicers, hot ovens, stoves, etc.

Prepares food for special events as requested.

Supervises kitchen personnel and coordinates their activities.

Prerequisites: Experience in large scale cooking.

Working Conditions:

Job Title: First Cook (Continued)

APPROVED:

____
Supervisor

____
Date

____
Department Head

____
Date

REVIEWED AND RETAINED:

____
Supervisor

____
Date

____
Department Head

____
Date

JOB TITLE: FIRST COOK DATE:

	BASIS OF EVALUATION	POINTS
SKILL	FACTOR #1 - MENTAL DEVELOPMENT -- Specific knowledge of large scale institutional cooking Benchmark Reference(s):	45
	FACTOR #2 - WORK EXPERIENCE -- Supervises entry level people in food preparation, must be proficient in all aspects Benchmark Reference(s):	45
	FACTOR #3 - JUDGMENT -- Must prepare menus as prescribed, solve kitchen problems Benchmark Reference(s):	20
RESPONSIBILITY	FACTOR #4 - ERRORS AND LOSSES -- Normal care required to assure food is prepared in accordance with recipes and in a sanitary and safe manner Benchmark Reference(s):	20
	FACTOR #5 - RESOURCE UTILIZATION -- Responsible for correct utilization of food and personnel Benchmark Reference(s):	30
	FACTOR #6 - SYSTEMS AND DATA -- Shares responsibility to deliver quality food on schedule Benchmark Reference(s):	30
	FACTOR #7 - INTERPERSONAL RELATIONSHIPS -- Directs activities of kitchen workers, some contacts with vendors and delivery Benchmark Reference(s):	30
WORKING CONDITIONS	FACTOR #8 - WORK ENVIRONMENT -- Exposure to steam, heat, dampness Benchmark Reference(s):	20
	FACTOR #9 - HAZARDS -- Subject to burns and cuts Benchmark Reference(s):	15
EFFORT	FACTOR #10 - PERSONAL DEMANDS -- Must stand all day, requires heavy lifting Benchmark Reference(s):	30

TOTAL POINT EVALUATION: 285

JOB DESCRIPTION

Job Title: Staff Dietitian

Department: Dietetic

Primary Function: Provides technical guidance and administrative direction over diet planning, menu formulation and the preparation and serving of foods.

Reports To (Title):

Supervises (Title):

Typical Duties: Assists in all duties concerning patient nutritional care.

Reviews physician's orders for modified diets and formulates menus for therapeutic and special diets.

Instructs patients in the proper procedure for making menus and reviews and modifies menus after selections have been made if needed.

Instructs patients and/or their relatives regarding diet therapy to be applied after discharge.

Interviews patients to obtain information regarding food habits and preferences, and to instruct regarding therapeutic diet.

Advises patient on types and quantities of food prescribed on therapeutic diet.

Supervises the tabulation of orders from menus and preparation of daily production sheets by cooks and production workers.

Assists in the supervision of tray and nourishment preparation according to established procedures and standards.

Records nutritional care on patient charts.

Prerequisites: Bachelor's degree with a major in foods and nutrition. Completion of a dietetic internship approved by the American Dietetic Association--ADA registration.

Job Title: Staff Dietitian (Continued)

Working Conditions:

APPROVED:

____
Supervisor

____
Date

____
Department Head

____
Date

REVIEWED AND RETAINED:

____
Supervisor

____
Date

____
Department Head

____
Date

JOB TITLE: STAFF DIETITIAN DATE:

	BASIS OF EVALUATION	POINTS
SKILL	FACTOR #1 - MENTAL DEVELOPMENT -- Specific knowledge of the principles of a specialized field and their application Benchmark Reference(s):	60
	FACTOR #2 - WORK EXPERIENCE -- Proficiency in administrative and therapeutic procedures, supervises diet clerks Benchmark Reference(s):	45
	FACTOR #3 - JUDGMENT -- Follows professional practices, creative diet planning necessary Benchmark Reference(s):	40
RESPONSIBILITY	FACTOR #4 - ERRORS AND LOSSES -- Considerable care to assure proper diet planned for patient Benchmark Reference(s):	30
	FACTOR #5 - RESOURCE UTILIZATION -- Supervises a section of dietary clerks Benchmark Reference(s):	30
	FACTOR #6 - SYSTEMS AND DATA -- Works as part of food service team, shares responsibility for nourishing food delivery Benchmark Reference(s):	30
	FACTOR #7 - INTERPERSONAL RELATIONSHIPS -- Interacts with patients, families, doctors, to explain diet needs Benchmark Reference(s):	60
WORKING CONDITIONS	FACTOR #8 - WORK ENVIRONMENT -- Comfortable conditions Benchmark Reference(s):	10
	FACTOR #9 - HAZARDS -- Occasional abuse from patients dissatisfied with menu Benchmark Reference(s):	10
EFFORT	FACTOR #10 - PERSONAL DEMANDS -- Close attention required to assure proper diet planning Benchmark Reference(s):	20

TOTAL POINT EVALUATION: 335

JOB DESCRIPTION

Job Title: Food Service Director

Department: Dietetic

Primary Function: Plans, directs and coordinates activities of the dietetics department to provide food and beverage service for patients, hospital employees, visitors, and special functions as requested.

Reports To (Title):

Supervises (Title):

Typical Duties: Supervises the dietary service for patients, cafeteria, and/or restaurant in accordance with departmental regulations, procedures, and hospital administrative policies.

Establishes regulations, departmental policies and procedures and inspects all work, storage and serving areas to determine compliance.

Ensures the preparation of quality food which meets the nutritional and therapeutic needs of the patients and, in addition, ensures all food is flavorful, served attractively, and at the proper temperature.

Maintains, evaluates and updates tested recipes and plans menus with the assistance of dietitians.

Determines quantity of food required, and may select and purchase perishables.

Ensures sanitary conditions in the storage, preparation, and serving areas as well as distribution and cleanup.

Determines kinds and amounts of supplies and equipment needed for efficient food preparation.

Maintains effective relationships with medical staff and other patient care services and confers with them regarding technical and administrative aspects of dietary service.

Job Title: Food Service Director (Continued)

Typical Duties: Supervises the food planning, preparation, service, and cleanup for special functions.

Maintains and/or reviews reports covering such items as number and kinds of meals prepared, costs of raw food and labor, inventory and handling of equipment and supplies, and other related information.

Interviews and selects employees and reviews work schedules, assignments, and performance.

Keeps informed of new developments and trends in the field of food preparation and suggests and implements improvements to hospital food service.

Handles patient and employee complaints regarding food service or preparation.

Prerequisites: Bachelor's degree with a major in foods, nutrition, or food service administration or experience in restraurant management.

Working Conditions:

APPROVED:	REVIEWED AND RETAINED:
______________________ Supervisor	______________________ Supervisor
______________________ Date	______________________ Date
______________________ Department Head	______________________ Department Head
______________________ Date	______________________ Date

JOB TITLE: FOOD SERVICE DIRECTOR DATE:

	BASIS OF EVALUATION	POINTS
SKILL	FACTOR #1 - MENTAL DEVELOPMENT -- Specific knowledge of the principles of a recognized field and their application Benchmark Reference(s):	60
	FACTOR #2 - WORK EXPERIENCE -- Requires proficiency in supervision - must be able to supervise many levels of personnel Benchmark Reference(s):	60
	FACTOR #3 - JUDGMENT -- Professional standards, must coordinate all facilities Benchmark Reference(s):	40
RESPONSIBILITY	FACTOR #4 - ERRORS AND LOSSES -- Constant care required to assure nutritious food delivered on a timely basis - responsible for adherence to safety and sanitary requirements Benchmark Reference(s):	40
	FACTOR #5 - RESOURCE UTILIZATION -- Responsible for purchasing, considerable staff costs, expensive equipment Benchmark Reference(s):	40
	FACTOR #6 - SYSTEMS AND DATA -- Responsible for preparation and delivery of food to patients and cafeteria Benchmark Reference(s):	40
	FACTOR #7 - INTERPERSONAL RELATIONSHIPS -- Coordinates activities of the department with needs of rest of hospital Benchmark Reference(s):	60
WORKING CONDITIONS	FACTOR #8 - WORK ENVIRONMENT -- Comfortable conditions - irregular hours Benchmark Reference(s):	10
	FACTOR #9 - HAZARDS -- Frequent minor abuse regarding menu selection Benchmark Reference(s):	10
EFFORT	FACTOR #10 - PERSONAL DEMANDS -- Considerable mental effort to coordinate and manage department Benchmark Reference(s):	30

TOTAL POINT EVALUATION: 390

JOB DESCRIPTION

Job Title: Dietary Clerk

Department: Dietetic

Primary Function: Performs a variety of clerical activities for the dietetic department.

Reports To (Title):

Supervises (Title):

Typical Duties: Compiles information used by kitchen personnel in preparation of food.

Tallies portions and kinds of food required and summarizes information on master menu.

Keeps records and prepares reports on such things as total meals served, food purchases, food costs, and inventory.

Inventories supplies and equipment.

Processes new diets and changes as required.

Answers phone and types requisitions for supplies.

Answers phone and takes requests for late trays and special diets.

Prerequisites: None

Working Conditions:

Job Title: Dietary Clerk (Continued)

APPROVED:

Supervisor

Date

Department Head

Date

REVIEWED AND RETAINED:

Supervisor

Date

Department Head

Date

JOB TITLE: DIETARY CLERK DATE:

	BASIS OF EVALUATION	POINTS
SKILL	FACTOR #1 - MENTAL DEVELOPMENT -- No specialized knowledge required Benchmark Reference(s):	15
	FACTOR #2 - WORK EXPERIENCE -- Must be able to recognize special diets, on-the-job training required Benchmark Reference(s):	30
	FACTOR #3 - JUDGMENT -- Some judgment required, must coordinate special diets or requests Benchmark Reference(s):	20
RESPONSIBILITY	FACTOR #4 - ERRORS AND LOSSES -- Normal care required to assure accurate reports and inventory counts Benchmark Reference(s):	20
	FACTOR #5 - RESOURCE UTILIZATION -- Reports impact for hospital resource planning Benchmark Reference(s):	20
	FACTOR #6 - SYSTEMS AND DATA -- Performs necessary paperwork to keep food system working Benchmark Reference(s):	20
	FACTOR #7 - INTERPERSONAL RELATIONSHIPS -- Takes requests Benchmark Reference(s):	15
WORKING CONDITIONS	FACTOR #8 - WORK ENVIRONMENT -- Next to kitchen Benchmark Reference(s):	10
	FACTOR #9 - HAZARDS -- Normal office environment Benchmark Reference(s):	5
EFFORT	FACTOR #10 - PERSONAL DEMANDS -- Requires close attention to assure accurate reports Benchmark Reference(s):	20
	TOTAL POINT EVALUATION:	175

JOB DESCRIPTION

Job Title:	Executive Housekeeper
Department:	Housekeeping
Primary Function:	Directs and administers the housekeeping program of the hospital to ensure it is maintained in an orderly and sanitary condition.
Reports To (Title):	
Supervises (Title):	
Typical Duties:	Establishes standards and housekeeping work procedures for all areas of the hospital staff. Plans work schedules and daily work assignments to ensure adequate cleaning. Interviews, hires and evaluates housekeeping personnel. Directs the training programs for all housekeeping personnel. Orders all supplies and reviews expenditures to comply with budget. Consults with other hospital departments to gather information required for planning and corrective action. Evaluates new products and cleaning methods and incorporates desirable changes into practice. Keeps department records and statistical data and submits repair requests to Plant Engineer.
Prerequisites:	Special courses in housekeeping or institutional management desired. Experience required as housekeeping supervisor.
Working Conditions:	

Job Title: Executive Housekeeper

APPROVED:	REVIEWED AND RETAINED:
______________________	______________________
Supervisor	Supervisor
______________________	______________________
Date	Date
______________________	______________________
Department Head	Department Head
______________________	______________________
Date	Date

JOB TITLE: EXECUTIVE HOUSEKEEPER DATE:

	BASIS OF EVALUATION	POINTS
SKILL	FACTOR #1 - MENTAL DEVELOPMENT -- Must know institutional cleaning policies, procedures and sanitary guidelines Benchmark Reference(s):	45
	FACTOR #2 - WORK EXPERIENCE -- Supervises a large number of personnel engaged in various tasks Benchmark Reference(s):	60
	FACTOR #3 - JUDGMENT -- Spends a lot of time problem solving and decision making Benchmark Reference(s):	40
RESPONSIBILITY	FACTOR #4 - ERRORS AND LOSSES -- Considerable care is required to assure compliance with sanitary regulations Benchmark Reference(s):	30
	FACTOR #5 - RESOURCE UTILIZATION -- Responsible for the resources and personnel of the department Benchmark Reference(s):	40
	FACTOR #6 - SYSTEMS AND DATA -- Responsible for clean conditions in entire hospital Benchmark Reference(s):	40
	FACTOR #7 - INTERPERSONAL RELATIONSHIPS -- Requires supervisory responsibility, coordinates activities with other areas Benchmark Reference(s):	45
WORKING CONDITIONS	FACTOR #8 - WORK ENVIRONMENT -- Comfortable conditions, irregular hours Benchmark Reference(s):	10
	FACTOR #9 - HAZARDS -- Accountable to patients, public and hospital staff regarding questions of service Benchmark Reference(s):	15
EFFORT	FACTOR #10 - PERSONAL DEMANDS -- Considerable effort to manage housekeeping function Benchmark Reference(s):	30

TOTAL POINT EVALUATION: 355

JOB DESCRIPTION

Job Title: Housekeeping Aide

Department: Housekeeping

Primary Function: Maintains an assigned area of the hospital in a clean, orderly, and sanitary condition.

Reports To (Title):

Supervises (Title):

Typical Duties:

Cleans assigned area by washing floors, furniture, and equipment with special cleaning solutions.

Vacuums carpeted areas and vents.

Empties containers such as ashtrays and trash baskets.

Arranges furniture in prescribed fashion.

Cleans restrooms by scouring fixtures and replenishes soap, towels and other dispensable items.

Reports mechanical failures and need for supplies to supervisor.

Makes beds with clean linen and removes soiled linen and trash to designated location.

Damp mop or wash areas such as walls, baseboards, windows and doors.

Prerequisites: None

Working Conditions:

Job Title: Housekeeping Aide (Continued)

APPROVED:	REVIEWED AND RETAINED:
______________________	______________________
Supervisor	Supervisor
______________________	______________________
Date	Date
______________________	______________________
Department Head	Department Head
______________________	______________________
Date	Date

JOB TITLE: HOUSEKEEPING AIDE DATE:

	BASIS OF EVALUATION	POINTS
SKILL	FACTOR #1 - MENTAL DEVELOPMENT -- No special knowledge required Benchmark Reference(s):	15
	FACTOR #2 - WORK EXPERIENCE -- On-the-job indoctrination Benchmark Reference(s):	15
	FACTOR #3 - JUDGMENT -- Routine work Benchmark Reference(s):	10
RESPONSIBILITY	FACTOR #4 - ERRORS AND LOSSES -- Closely supervised; supervisor responsible for errors Benchmark Reference(s):	10
	FACTOR #5 - RESOURCE UTILIZATION -- Use of supplies controlled Benchmark Reference(s):	10
	FACTOR #6 - SYSTEMS AND DATA -- Works as part of team Benchmark Reference(s):	20
	FACTOR #7 - INTERPERSONAL RELATIONSHIPS -- Limited contacts with patients, other departments Benchmark Reference(s):	15
WORKING CONDITIONS	FACTOR #8 - WORK ENVIRONMENT -- Regular exposure to disagreeable work elements, chemicals, dirt, noise (vacuum) Benchmark Reference(s):	15
	FACTOR #9 - HAZARDS -- Cuts, bruises possible Benchmark Reference(s):	15
EFFORT	FACTOR #10 - PERSONAL DEMANDS -- Constantly on feet, scrubbing, lifting garbage Benchmark Reference(s):	30

TOTAL POINT EVALUATION: 155

JOB DESCRIPTION

Job Title: Housekeeping Supervisor

Department: Housekeeping

Primary Function: Supervises all housekeeping personnel to ensure that a clean and attractive hospital environment is maintained.

Reports To (Title):

Supervises (Title):

Typical Duties:

Supervises and maintains the flow of work for all housekeeping employees and checks quality and quantity of work performed.

Ensures that all areas have adequate supplies and staff and delivers supplies to working areas.

Maintains absenteeism records and other personnel data.

Completes work requisitions for any maintenance repairs.

Trains new employees and closely supervises their activities until fully trained.

Instructs personnel on use of new equipment or new cleaning methods.

Maintains records of rooms and hospital areas that have been cleared and rooms ready for new occupancy.

Ensures garbage and trash disposal meet safety and health regulations.

Makes recommendations for personnel actions such as hiring, terminating and transferring.

Prerequisites: Experience in housekeeping procedures and knowledge of sanitary regulations.

Job Title: Housekeeping Supervisor (Continued)

Working Conditions:

APPROVED:	REVIEWED AND RETAINED:
______________________ Supervisor	______________________ Supervisor
______________________ Date	______________________ Date
______________________ Department Head	______________________ Department Head
______________________ Date	______________________ Date

JOB TITLE: HOUSEKEEPING SUPERVISOR DATE:

	BASIS OF EVALUATION	POINTS
SKILL	FACTOR #1 - MENTAL DEVELOPMENT -- Must know cleaning agencies, housekeeping techniques Benchmark Reference(s):	30
	FACTOR #2 - WORK EXPERIENCE -- Must be able to train housekeepers in all duties Benchmark Reference(s):	45
	FACTOR #3 - JUDGMENT -- Work load given, some judgment in assigning tasks Benchmark Reference(s):	20
RESPONSIBILITY	FACTOR #4 - ERRORS AND LOSSES -- Care to avoid error to reduce complaints and sanitary problems Benchmark Reference(s):	20
	FACTOR #5 - RESOURCE UTILIZATION -- Must train in effective and efficient use of housekeeping supplies, responsible for efficient use of personnel Benchmark Reference(s):	20
	FACTOR #6 - SYSTEMS AND DATA -- Supervises housekeeping process in assigned areas Benchmark Reference(s):	30
	FACTOR #7 - INTERPERSONAL RELATIONSHIPS -- Coordinates activities with admitting, nursing service, etc. Benchmark Reference(s):	30
WORKING CONDITIONS	FACTOR #8 - WORK ENVIRONMENT -- Regular exposure to disagreeable elements Benchmark Reference(s):	15
	FACTOR #9 - HAZARDS -- Some exposure to hazards, some stress in supervision Benchmark Reference(s):	10
EFFORT	FACTOR #10 - PERSONAL DEMANDS -- Constant standing and walking Benchmark Reference(s):	20

TOTAL POINT EVALUATION: 240

JOB DESCRIPTION

Job Title: Security Guard

Department: Plant Engineering

Primary Function: Patrols hospital buildings and grounds to enforce hospital safety and security and control hospital traffic and parking. Stands guard to maintain security at key access points.

Reports To (Title):

Supervises (Title):

Typical Duties:

Patrols indoors and outdoors to ensure that security standards are met and maintained.

Confronts unauthorized persons.

Enforces hospital security, traffic, and parking policies and procedures.

Controls parking and traffic to provide orderly traffic flow.

Observes and reports unsafe conditions.

Assists visitors entering and leaving the hospital.

Escorts female personnel to and from vehicles during hours of darkness.

Checks all key stations and other designated areas to detect security violations.

Inspects unauthorized parcels leaving the hospital.

Sounds fire signal and alerts fire department in the event of fire, and assists in extinguishing fire.

Prerequisites: None

Working Conditions:

Job Title: Security Guard (Continued)

APPROVED:

____
Supervisor

____
Date

____
Department Head

____
Date

REVIEWED AND RETAINED:

____
Supervisor

____
Date

____
Department Head

____
Date

JOB TITLE: SECURITY GUARD DATE:

	BASIS OF EVALUATION	POINTS
SKILL	FACTOR #1 - MENTAL DEVELOPMENT -- No specialized knowledge required Benchmark Reference(s):	15
	FACTOR #2 - WORK EXPERIENCE -- Must learn hospital procedures, routine Benchmark Reference(s):	30
	FACTOR #3 - JUDGMENT -- Judgment required to solve specific problems Benchmark Reference(s):	30
RESPONSIBILITY	FACTOR #4 - ERRORS AND LOSSES -- Normal care required in inspection activities Benchmark Reference(s):	20
	FACTOR #5 - RESOURCE UTILIZATION -- Protects hospital resources Benchmark Reference(s):	20
	FACTOR #6 - SYSTEMS AND DATA -- Discretion required in handling security matters Benchmark Reference(s):	20
	FACTOR #7 - INTERPERSONAL RELATIONSHIPS -- May confront visitors or employees, assists employees in emergencies Benchmark Reference(s):	30
WORKING CONDITIONS	FACTOR #8 - WORK ENVIRONMENT -- Comfortable conditions, outside periodically, irregular hours Benchmark Reference(s):	10
	FACTOR #9 - HAZARDS -- Occasional minor abuse Benchmark Reference(s):	10
EFFORT	FACTOR #10 - PERSONAL DEMANDS -- Standing and walking, must be alert at all times Benchmark Reference(s):	20

TOTAL POINT EVALUATION: 205

JOB DESCRIPTION

Job Title: Maintenance Mechanic

Department: Plant Engineering

Primary Function: Performs a variety of duties in the maintenance and repair of hospital facilities and equipment.

Reports To (Title):

Supervises (Title):

Typical Duties:

Performs a wide array of assigned general repairs and replaces defective parts on such items as wall sockets, switches, lamps, beds, bed controls, and makes minor adjustments on televisions.

Installs, maintains, and repairs mechanical devices such as pumps, motors, conveyor systems, laboratory equipment, air conditioning, refrigeration, and air handling equipment and controls.

Replaces light bulbs and fluorescent lights.

Repairs dressers, cabinets and tables.

Carries out preventative maintenance program and keeps associated records.

Operates hand and power tools and precision measuring instruments.

Assists in maintaining uninterrupted, efficient and safe operation of heating, ventilation and air conditioning systems.

Documents work completed and time required as part of work order system and time recording requirements.

Initiates requests for purchasing requisitions to obtain materials necessary to perform repairs or alterations.

Paints or wallpapers rooms, hallways, ceilings, etc., as required.

<u>Job Title</u>: Maintenance Mechanic (Continued)

<u>Typical Duties</u>: Assists in performing plumbing and steamfitting duties required for maintaining continuity of service.

<u>Prerequisites</u>: Demonstrates a good knowledge of mechanical systems and their repair and maintenance.

<u>Working Conditions</u>:

APPROVED:	REVIEWED AND RETAINED:
Supervisor	Supervisor
Date	Date
Department Head	Department Head
Date	Date

JOB TITLE: MAINTENANCE MECHANIC DATE:

	BASIS OF EVALUATION	POINTS
SKILL	FACTOR #1 - MENTAL DEVELOPMENT -- Must have general knowledge of mechanical systems and their maintenance Benchmark Reference(s):	30
	FACTOR #2 - WORK EXPERIENCE -- Must know how to repair many types of machines and equipment Benchmark Reference(s):	45
	FACTOR #3 - JUDGMENT -- Uses standard practice, solves specific repair problems Benchmark Reference(s):	30
RESPONSIBILITY	FACTOR #4 - ERRORS AND LOSSES -- Requires considerable care to assure repairs performed in a safe and reliable manner. Benchmark Reference(s):	30
	FACTOR #5 - RESOURCE UTILIZATION -- Uses tools and supplies in repairs Benchmark Reference(s):	20
	FACTOR #6 - SYSTEMS AND DATA -- Works as part of team; other mechanics may be able to cover Benchmark Reference(s):	20
	FACTOR #7 - INTERPERSONAL RELATIONSHIPS -- Communicates with other employees in making repairs Benchmark Reference(s):	30
WORKING CONDITIONS	FACTOR #8 - WORK ENVIRONMENT -- Continuous exposure to disagreeable work conditions Benchmark Reference(s):	20
	FACTOR #9 - HAZARDS -- Regular exposure to hazards Benchmark Reference(s):	15
EFFORT	FACTOR #10 - PERSONAL DEMANDS -- Considerable physical effort, awkward positions, etc. Benchmark Reference(s):	30

TOTAL POINT EVALUATION: 270

JOB DESCRIPTION

Job Title: Maintenance Supervisor

Department: Plant Engineering

Primary Function: Supervises and assigns work to maintenance personnel in the routine maintenance and repair of building, grounds and utilities and assists in establishing regular maintenance schedules for all major equipment.

Reports to (Title):

Supervises (Title):

Typical Duties: Receives repair orders from various departments, establishes priorities and determines work schedules.

Requisitions supplies, materials, parts and equipment as needed.

Assists in computing and controlling repair costs for budgeting purposes and maintains appropriate records.

Provides technical assistance to maintenance personnel in performance of repairs and maintenance as required.

Assists in interviewing, selecting and training new maintenance personnel.

Maintains appropriate records to log maintenance and repair activities.

Performs any of the duties of a maintenance mechanic as workload requires.

Assures that workmanship meets hospital and state safety guidelines.

Prerequisites: Demonstrates a sound knowledge of maintenance and repair procedures for a wide variety of hospital equipment, utilities and building problems.

Job Title: Maintenance Supervisor (Continued)

Working Conditions:

APPROVED:	REVIEWED AND RETAINED:
______________________	______________________
Supervisor	Supervisor
______________________	______________________
Date	Date
______________________	______________________
Department Head	Department Head
______________________	______________________
Date	Date

JOB TITLE: MAINTENANCE SUPERVISOR DATE:

	BASIS OF EVALUATION	POINTS
SKILL	FACTOR #1 - MENTAL DEVELOPMENT -- Must have sound knowledge of repair procedures for a wide variety of hospital equipment, utilities Benchmark Reference(s):	45
	FACTOR #2 - WORK EXPERIENCE -- Must train and supervise mechanics in numerous repair procedures Benchmark Reference(s):	60
	FACTOR #3 - JUDGMENT -- Works according to established procedures Benchmark Reference(s):	30
RESPONSIBILITY	FACTOR #4 - ERRORS AND LOSSES -- Considerable care to assure preventative maintenance done, repairs done in safe manner Benchmark Reference(s):	30
	FACTOR #5 - RESOURCE UTILIZATION -- Responsible for section or group, costs repair jobs Benchmark Reference(s):	30
	FACTOR #6 - SYSTEMS AND DATA -- Work leader - must assure repairs done on timely basis Benchmark Reference(s):	30
	FACTOR #7 - INTERPERSONAL RELATIONSHIPS -- Supervisor - contacts with other departments regarding repairs Benchmark Reference(s):	45
WORKING CONDITIONS	FACTOR #8 - WORK ENVIRONMENT -- Regular exposure to disagreeable elements Benchmark Reference(s):	15
	FACTOR #9 - HAZARDS -- Exposure to disagreeable elements when assisting mechanics Benchmark Reference(s):	10
EFFORT	FACTOR #10 - PERSONAL DEMANDS -- Constant standing, walking, supervisory stress Benchmark Reference(s):	20
	TOTAL POINT EVALUATION:	315

JOB DESCRIPTION

Job Title: Plant Operations Manager

Department: Plant Engineering

Primary Function: Organizes, plans, directs, and administers programs to develop and maintain hospital buildings, facilities and equipment, and is responsible for maintaining a comfortable, safe, and efficient physical environment.

Reports To (Title):

Supervises (Title):

Typical Duties: Ensures hospital compliance with all local, state, federal, and Joint Commission regulations and codes pertaining to physical environment.

Plans and recommends enhancement of physical facilities and advises administration and planning department regarding structural changes and acceptance of contract bids.

Negotiates with outside contractors for remodeling, repairs and installations to buildings, grounds and coordinates services provided by outside contractors with other hospital departments.

Initiates, develops and directs implementation of plant operating policies and maintenance procedures for preventative maintenance; appraises policies for maximum operating efficiency.

Informs administration of current plant and department status and prepares required reports for both in and outside the hospital.

Analyzes cost and work schedules; sets priorities; expedites operations and repairs.

Periodically inspects buildings and utility systems to assure compliance with safety guidelines.

Monitors cost of plant operations and approves requisitions for equipment and supplies.

Job Title: Plant Operations Manager (Continued)

Typical Duties:

Maintains preventive maintenance program, sets quality standards and inspects for compliance.

Participates in committee functions as assigned, i.e., infection control, safety, etc.

Serves as Fire Marshall and as such inspects and monitors fire equipment and ensures that training sessions on fire procedures and prevention for all hospital employees are conducted.

Schedules, supervises, assigns, and evaluates department personnel.

Interviews prospective department employees, makes recommendations of hire, and listens to employees' suggestions and grievances.

Reviews all department reports and correspondence for compliance with operating and maintenance policies.

Participates in associations, technical, and civic groups related to plant operation and keeps informed of new and improved materials, equipment and methods, and their application to the hospital.

Prerequisites: Bachelor of Science in mechanical or electrical engineering. Demonstrates a thorough knowledge of hospital plant facilities and their maintenance.

Working Conditions:

APPROVED:	REVIEWED AND RETAINED:
Supervisor	Supervisor
Date	Date
Department Head	Department Head
Date	Date

JOB TITLE: PLANT OPERATIONS MANAGER　　　　DATE:

	BASIS OF EVALUATION	POINTS
SKILL	FACTOR #1 - MENTAL DEVELOPMENT -- Must have engineering background, be able to apply principles Benchmark Reference(s):	60
	FACTOR #2 - WORK EXPERIENCE -- Must have a thorough knowledge of hospital plant facilities, maintenance and related regulations Benchmark Reference(s):	75
	FACTOR #3 - JUDGMENT -- Majority of time spent in planning and coordinating activities Benchmark Reference(s):	40
RESPONSIBILITY	FACTOR #4 - ERRORS AND LOSSES -- Requires extreme care to assure safe and effective environment properly maintained Benchmark Reference(s):	50
	FACTOR #5 - RESOURCE UTILIZATION -- Maintain expensive hospital equipment and facilities constituting a major component of financial resources Benchmark Reference(s):	50
	FACTOR #6 - SYSTEMS AND DATA -- Responsible for all maintenance systems Benchmark Reference(s):	50
	FACTOR #7 - INTERPERSONAL RELATIONSHIPS -- Supervises diverse activities, coordinates with outside contractors and departments Benchmark Reference(s):	60
WORKING CONDITIONS	FACTOR #8 - WORK ENVIRONMENT -- Some exposure to disagreeable conditions Benchmark Reference(s):	10
	FACTOR #9 - HAZARDS -- May receive minor abuse from staff regarding repairs Benchmark Reference(s):	10
EFFORT	FACTOR #10 - PERSONAL DEMANDS -- Stress in managing department Benchmark Reference(s):	30

TOTAL POINT EVALUATION: 435

JOB DESCRIPTION

Job Title: Purchasing Agent

Department: Purchasing and Receiving

Primary Function: Carries out varied purchasing assignments requiring negotiation with vendors. Exercises judgment in selection of supply source based on good working knowledge of materials to be purchased.

Reports to (Title):

Supervises (Title):

Typical Duties: Assists in establishing procedures for receiving, storing, and issuing purchased items.

Reviews inventory of stock items and initiates purchasing of medical equipment, furnishings, supplies and building materials within established guidelines.

Compares prices, specifications, and delivery dates on items of purchase of various vendors and recommends new vendors as warranted.

Consults with department heads to determine the quality, effectiveness, and durability of products purchased.

Compiles and prepares monthly reports on major purchases for inventory and budget purposes.

Prerequisites: Demonstrates a good knowledge of purchasing policies and procedures and hospital equipment and supplies.

Working Conditions:

Job Title: Purchasing Agent (Continued)

APPROVED:	REVIEWED AND RETAINED:
______________________	______________________
Supervisor	Supervisor
______________________	______________________
Date	Date
______________________	______________________
Department Head	Department Head
______________________	______________________
Date	Date

JOB TITLE: PURCHASING AGENT DATE:

	BASIS OF EVALUATION	POINTS
SKILL	FACTOR #1 - MENTAL DEVELOPMENT -- Must have a good knowledge of purchasing policies, procedures, hospital equipment and supplies Benchmark Reference(s):	45
	FACTOR #2 - WORK EXPERIENCE -- Must have knowledge of offices, equipment and supplies Benchmark Reference(s):	45
	FACTOR #3 - JUDGMENT -- Standard practice followed, may have to make substitutions Benchmark Reference(s):	30
RESPONSIBILITY	FACTOR #4 - ERRORS AND LOSSES -- Requires considerable care to verify invoices and monitor inventory levels Benchmark Reference(s):	30
	FACTOR #5 - RESOURCE UTILIZATION -- Controls ordering of supplies Benchmark Reference(s):	30
	FACTOR #6 - SYSTEMS AND DATA -- Must set up systems to monitor inventory levels and assure they are at accurate levels Benchmark Reference(s):	30
	FACTOR #7 - INTERPERSONAL RELATIONSHIPS -- Confers with vendors, negotiates prices and delivery dates Benchmark Reference(s):	45
WORKING CONDITIONS	FACTOR #8 - WORK ENVIRONMENT -- Office environment Benchmark Reference(s):	5
	FACTOR #9 - HAZARDS -- Occasional abuse regarding supply levels Benchmark Reference(s):	10
EFFORT	FACTOR #10 - PERSONAL DEMANDS -- Close attention when ordering and verifying invoices Benchmark Reference(s):	20

TOTAL POINT EVALUATION: 290

JOB DESCRIPTION

Job Title: PBX/Switchboard Operator

Department: Financial Management

Primary Function: Operates telephone console, answers and routes in-house and incoming telephone calls; processes and records charges on patient and hospital personnel long-distance calls and pages doctors and other hospital personnel as required.

Reports To (Title):

Supervises (Title):

Typical Duties: Answers and routes incoming telephone calls to proper patient and/or hospital personnel.

Answers and routes in-house calls.

Processes patient and hospital personnel long-distance calls, records same and posts charges.

Responds to medical, fire and disaster emergency situations by notifying appropriate personnel.

Answers ambulance-to-hospital radio calls, receives and routes patient information.

Prerequisites: None

Working Conditions:

APPROVED:	REVIEWED AND RETAINED:
Supervisor	Supervisor
Date	Date
Department Head	Department Head
Date	Date

JOB TITLE: PBX/SWITCHBOARD OPERATOR DATE:

	BASIS OF EVALUATION	POINTS
SKILL	FACTOR #1 - MENTAL DEVELOPMENT -- No specialized knowledge required Benchmark Reference(s):	15
	FACTOR #2 - WORK EXPERIENCE -- Must be trained to handle emergencies Benchmark Reference(s):	30
	FACTOR #3 - JUDGMENT -- Detailed job procedures, some room for judgment Benchmark Reference(s):	20
RESPONSIBILITY	FACTOR #4 - ERRORS AND LOSSES -- Normal care required to accurately transfer calls Benchmark Reference(s):	20
	FACTOR #5 - RESOURCE UTILIZATION -- Limited effect on the hospital resources Benchmark Reference(s):	10
	FACTOR #6 - SYSTEMS AND DATA -- Works as part of a team, uses discretion in handling information Benchmark Reference(s):	20
	FACTOR #7 - INTERPERSONAL RELATIONSHIPS -- Frequent contacts with outside callers Benchmark Reference(s):	30
WORKING CONDITIONS	FACTOR #8 - WORK ENVIRONMENT -- Some disagreeable elements confined to telephone console Benchmark Reference(s):	10
	FACTOR #9 - HAZARDS -- Occasional minor abuse from callers Benchmark Reference(s):	10
EFFORT	FACTOR #10 - PERSONAL DEMANDS -- Normal work place attention Benchmark Reference(s):	10

TOTAL POINT EVALUATION: 175

JOB DESCRIPTION

Job Title: Payroll Clerk

Department: Financial Management

Primary Function: Computes and processes payroll information and records in keeping with established hospital policy and procedure, and performs a variety of other clerical services.

Reports To (Title):

Supervises (Title):

Typical Duties:

Processes time cards by computing hours worked for each payroll.

Computes deductions such as income tax, withholding, social security payments, insurance, etc.

Posts information on control sheets.

Transmits payroll information to payroll check preparers.

Maintains records of sick time, vacation or other leave.

Answers questions regarding employee's paycheck amounts.

Maintains records concerning retirement and insurance renewals and terminations.

Prerequisites: Successful completion of on-the-job training.

Working Conditions:

Job Title: Payroll Clerk (Continued)

APPROVED:	REVIEWED AND RETAINED:
______________________	______________________
Supervisor	Supervisor
______________________	______________________
Date	Date
______________________	______________________
Department Head	Department Head
______________________	______________________
Date	Date

JOB TITLE: PAYROLL CLERK DATE:

	BASIS OF EVALUATION	POINTS
SKILL	FACTOR #1 - MENTAL DEVELOPMENT -- General knowledge of arithmetic and its application required Benchmark Reference(s):	30
	FACTOR #2 - WORK EXPERIENCE -- Must know hospital policies and procedures regarding vacation, overtime, compensatory time, deductions, taxation Benchmark Reference(s):	45
	FACTOR #3 - JUDGMENT -- Detailed work procedures, some judgment required in unusual problems Benchmark Reference(s):	20
RESPONSIBILITY	FACTOR #4 - ERRORS AND LOSSES -- Considerable care required to assure accurate paychecks, tax payments, etc. Benchmark Reference(s):	30
	FACTOR #5 - RESOURCE UTILIZATION -- Responsible for properly paying vacation, overtime, etc., as well as routine payroll Benchmark Reference(s):	30
	FACTOR #6 - SYSTEMS AND DATA -- Shares responsibility for a process, handles confidential information Benchmark Reference(s):	30
	FACTOR #7 - INTERPERSONAL RELATIONSHIPS -- Contacts with employees regarding payroll problems Benchmark Reference(s):	30
WORKING CONDITIONS	FACTOR #8 - WORK ENVIRONMENT -- Office conditions Benchmark Reference(s):	5
	FACTOR #9 - HAZARDS -- Occasional minor abuse regarding payroll errors Benchmark Reference(s):	10
EFFORT	FACTOR #10 - PERSONAL DEMANDS -- Close attention required Benchmark Reference(s):	20

TOTAL POINT EVALUATION: 250

JOB DESCRIPTION

Job Title: Admitting Clerk

Department: Financial Management

Primary Function: Assures accurate information on incoming patients through interviews with them or their representatives, records information required for admission, and assigns patient to a room.

Reports To (Title):

Supervises (Title):

Typical Duties:

Interviews patient or their representative to obtain identifying information, physician name, and insurance coverage data as per established guidelines.

Enters information onto appropriate forms.

Obtains patient signatures.

Prepares identification plates and arm bracelets.

Explains hospital procedures and rules to patients.

Stores patients' valuables in hospital vault.

Takes reservations for rooms, assigns patients to rooms, ensures that rooms are ready for patients.

Distributes admission forms to appropriate departments.

Makes necessary preadmission arrangements.

Performs miscellaneous other duties as assigned.

Prerequisites: None

Job Title: Admitting Clerk (Continued)

Working Conditions:

APPROVED:	REVIEWED AND RETAINED:
Supervisor	Supervisor
Date	Date
Department Head	Department Head
Date	Date

JOB TITLE: ADMITTING CLERK DATE:

	BASIS OF EVALUATION	POINTS
SKILL	FACTOR #1 - MENTAL DEVELOPMENT -- No specialized knowledge required Benchmark Reference(s):	15
SKILL	FACTOR #2 - WORK EXPERIENCE -- Basic on-the-job training Benchmark Reference(s):	30
SKILL	FACTOR #3 - JUDGMENT -- Some room for judgment Benchmark Reference(s):	20
RESPONSIBILITY	FACTOR #4 - ERRORS AND LOSSES -- Normal care required to avoid errors Benchmark Reference(s):	20
RESPONSIBILITY	FACTOR #5 - RESOURCE UTILIZATION -- Responsible for prompt admitting Benchmark Reference(s):	20
RESPONSIBILITY	FACTOR #6 - SYSTEMS AND DATA -- Works as part of a team, handles information which requires discretion Benchmark Reference(s):	20
RESPONSIBILITY	FACTOR #7 - INTERPERSONAL RELATIONSHIPS -- Continual and substantive contact with patients and public Benchmark Reference(s):	45
WORKING CONDITIONS	FACTOR #8 - WORK ENVIRONMENT -- Frequently noisy Benchmark Reference(s):	10
WORKING CONDITIONS	FACTOR #9 - HAZARDS -- Minor abuse from patients Benchmark Reference(s):	10
EFFORT	FACTOR #10 - PERSONAL DEMANDS -- Requires close attention to complete forms properly Benchmark Reference(s):	20

TOTAL POINT EVALUATION: 210

JOB DESCRIPTION

Job Title: Admitting Supervisor

Department: Financial Management

Primary Function: Supervises, coordinates and controls the activities of the hospital admitting office to arrange for patients' admission, transfer, discharge and future reservations.

Reports To (Title):

Supervises (Title):

Typical Duties: Supervises department personnel, ensures the proper and efficient admission of patients within hospital guidelines, and assists them in handling difficult or problem admissions.

Schedules admitting office personnel to ensure proper coverage.

Assists in interviewing and selecting and trains and instructs new department personnel.

Interviews patients or their representatives to obtain admission data, enters information onto forms and performs complete admission process.

Accepts reservations for future admissions and ensures bed availability.

Prepares census report and distributes.

Notifies nursing stations, housekeeping and other departments as required, of transfer room assignments.

Assists in emergency outpatient admissions.

Performs other related duties as required.

Prerequisites: Demonstrates a sound knowledge of admitting policies and procedures.

Job Title: Admitting Supervisor (Continued)

Working Conditions:

APPROVED:	REVIEWED AND RETAINED:
____________________ Supervisor	____________________ Supervisor
____________________ Date	____________________ Date
____________________ Department Head	____________________ Department Head
____________________ Date	____________________ Date

JOB TITLE: ADMITTING SUPERVISOR DATE:

	BASIS OF EVALUATION	POINTS
SKILL	FACTOR #1 - MENTAL DEVELOPMENT -- Must have a sound knowledge of admitting policies and procedures Benchmark Reference(s):	45
	FACTOR #2 - WORK EXPERIENCE -- Supervises and trains admitting clerks (proficiency required) Benchmark Reference(s):	45
	FACTOR #3 - JUDGMENT -- Follows standards, solves problems as they arise Benchmark Reference(s):	30
RESPONSIBILITY	FACTOR #4 - ERRORS AND LOSSES -- Assures that patients admitted correctly, proper information collected Benchmark Reference(s):	30
	FACTOR #5 - RESOURCE UTILIZATION -- Responsible for effective utilization of admitting clerks Benchmark Reference(s):	30
	FACTOR #6 - SYSTEMS AND DATA -- Responsible for keeping admitting process running smoothly Benchmark Reference(s):	40
	FACTOR #7 - INTERPERSONAL RELATIONSHIPS -- Supervisory responsibility, coordinates with other departments, deals with patient/admitting problems Benchmark Reference(s):	45
WORKING CONDITIONS	FACTOR #8 - WORK ENVIRONMENT -- Office conditions Benchmark Reference(s):	5
	FACTOR #9 - HAZARDS -- Abuse from public and hospital staff Benchmark Reference(s):	15
EFFORT	FACTOR #10 - PERSONAL DEMANDS -- Close attention to assure admitting process runs smoothly Benchmark Reference(s):	20

TOTAL POINT EVALUATION: 305

JOB DESCRIPTION

Job Title: Insurance Billing Clerk

Department: Financial Management

Primary Function: Determines financial responsibility of patient and various financial agencies for hospital charges; bills appropriate parties and follows up as required.

Reports To (Title):

Supervises (Title):

Typical Duties:

Codes patient files to reflect payment responsibilities based upon information provided by admitting office and insurance verification clerk.

Prepares and mails bills for patients and financing agencies.

Contacts financing agencies regarding past due claims to determine reasons.

Answers inquiries concerning accounts and documents above contacts.

Rebills appropriate parties for late charges or credits.

Substitutes in other business office positions as required.

Keeps abreast regarding insurance benefits and restrictions.

Prerequisites: Successful completion of on-the-job training.

Working Conditions:

Job Title: Insurance Billing Clerk (Continued)

APPROVED:	REVIEWED AND RETAINED:
______________________	______________________
Supervisor	Supervisor
______________________	______________________
Date	Date
______________________	______________________
Department Head	Department Head
______________________	______________________
Date	Date

JOB TITLE: INSURANCE BILLING CLERK DATE:

	BASIS OF EVALUATION	POINTS
SKILL	FACTOR #1 - MENTAL DEVELOPMENT -- Must be able to understand and apply Medicare and Medicaid coverages Benchmark Reference(s):	30
	FACTOR #2 - WORK EXPERIENCE -- On-the-job training required Benchmark Reference(s):	30
	FACTOR #3 - JUDGMENT -- Within standard practice, solves specific problems Benchmark Reference(s):	30
RESPONSIBILITY	FACTOR #4 - ERRORS AND LOSSES -- Considerable care required to assure proper allocation of bills and follow-up of payment Benchmark Reference(s):	30
	FACTOR #5 - RESOURCE UTILIZATION -- Follow-up to assure receipt of Medicare and Medicaid payments Benchmark Reference(s):	20
	FACTOR #6 - SYSTEMS AND DATA -- Works within Medicare, Medicaid Benchmark Reference(s):	20
	FACTOR #7 - INTERPERSONAL RELATIONSHIPS -- Confers with outside financial institutions regarding accounts Benchmark Reference(s):	30
WORKING CONDITIONS	FACTOR #8 - WORK ENVIRONMENT -- Office conditions Benchmark Reference(s):	5
	FACTOR #9 - HAZARDS -- Normal office routine Benchmark Reference(s):	5
EFFORT	FACTOR #10 - PERSONAL DEMANDS -- Close attention to assure accurate records Benchmark Reference(s):	20

TOTAL POINT EVALUATION: 220

JOB DESCRIPTION

Job Title: Accountant

Department: Financial Management

Primary Function: Maintains the general accounting system in the hospital by applying principles of accounting and statistical analysis and prepares various financial and budget reports.

Reports To (Title):

Supervises (Title):

Typical Duties: Coordinates and prepares financial and operating reports to reflect the financial condition of the hospital.

Prepares analyses of all general ledger accounts and suggests and implements systems and procedures for general accounting, payroll, accounts payable and receivable to improve operations.

Reviews and approves vouchers for payment. Assists the Comptroller in the preparation and interpretation of various budget reports. Evaluates subordinate activities.

Directs the activities of posting entries in ledgers such as accounts payable and receivable and resolves discrepancies.

Computes and files tax returns, patient welfare, and other insurance reports required by government agencies.

Audits cash receipts, disbursements, payroll, and time cards for accuracy.

Computes net income, expenses and profit/loss for each operating department.

Reviews incoming documents such as invoices, purchase orders, receiving documents, confirmation vouchers, requisitions and statements.

Responds to correspondence from suppliers, auditors, etc.

Job Title: Accountant (Continued)

Prerequisites: Bachelor's degree in Accounting.

Working Conditions:

APPROVED:	REVIEWED AND RETAINED:
______________________ Supervisor	______________________ Supervisor
______________________ Date	______________________ Date
______________________ Department Head	______________________ Department Head
______________________ Date	______________________ Date

JOB TITLE: ACCOUNTANT DATE:

	BASIS OF EVALUATION	POINTS
SKILL	FACTOR #1 - MENTAL DEVELOPMENT -- Must know generally accepted accounting principles and their applications Benchmark Reference(s):	60
	FACTOR #2 - WORK EXPERIENCE -- Must be proficient in hospital policies and procedures Benchmark Reference(s):	45
	FACTOR #3 - JUDGMENT -- Follows professional practices Benchmark Reference(s):	30
RESPONSIBILITY	FACTOR #4 - ERRORS AND LOSSES -- Constant care required in developing financial records, reports reviewed by controller Benchmark Reference(s):	40
	FACTOR #5 - RESOURCE UTILIZATION -- Directs accounting clerks, could have significant impact on financial records Benchmark Reference(s):	30
	FACTOR #6 - SYSTEMS AND DATA -- Shares responsibility of financial reporting process Benchmark Reference(s):	40
	FACTOR #7 - INTERPERSONAL RELATIONSHIPS -- Contacts with outside auditors, other departments. Supervises accounts payable clerks Benchmark Reference(s):	45
WORKING CONDITIONS	FACTOR #8 - WORK ENVIRONMENT -- Office conditions Benchmark Reference(s):	5
	FACTOR #9 - HAZARDS -- Must deal with financial problems and imbalances Benchmark Reference(s):	10
EFFORT	FACTOR #10 - PERSONAL DEMANDS -- Requires concentration on detailed reports and calculations Benchmark Reference(s):	30

TOTAL POINT EVALUATION: 335

JOB DESCRIPTION

Job Title: Business Office Supervisor

Department: Financial Management

Primary Function: Supervises and coordinates the activities of hospital Business Office personnel engaged in cashiering, insurance, telephone communications, credit and collections, reception and billing.

Reports To (Title):

Supervises (Title):

Typical Duties: Supervises clerical functions such as typing, bookkeeping, billing and other clerical service.

Develops business office procedures in compliance with hospital guidelines and initiates policy and procedural changes as required.

Develops, implements and evaluates clerical accounting and bookkeeping systems and controls. Subject to approvals to ensure an effective accounting for hospital revenues.

Requisitions office supplies and equipment, adhering to approved unit budget.

Assures that outstanding accounts receivable are reviewed and that collection is attempted.

Supervises collection and receipt of all in-patient revenue.

Reviews clerical and personnel records to ensure completness, accuracy and timeliness.

Prerequisites: Demonstrates a sound knowledge of cashiering, insurance, credit, collection and billing functions.

Working Conditions:

Job Title: Business Office Supervisor (Continued)

APPROVED:	REVIEWED AND RETAINED:
Supervisor	Supervisor
Date	Date
Department Head	Department Head
Date	Date

JOB TITLE: BUSINESS OFFICE SUPERVISOR DATE:

	BASIS OF EVALUATION	POINTS
SKILL	FACTOR #1 - MENTAL DEVELOPMENT -- Must know credit, collections, billing and insurance principles and practices Benchmark Reference(s):	45
	FACTOR #2 - WORK EXPERIENCE -- Must be familiar with and train and supervise in all business office functions Benchmark Reference(s):	60
	FACTOR #3 - JUDGMENT -- Follows professional business practices, spends majority of time in decision making Benchmark Reference(s):	40
RESPONSIBILITY	FACTOR #4 - ERRORS AND LOSSES -- Constant care required to assure accurate billing and reporting Benchmark Reference(s):	40
	FACTOR #5 - RESOURCE UTILIZATION -- Responsible for effective utilization of business office staff Benchmark Reference(s):	40
	FACTOR #6 - SYSTEMS AND DATA -- Responsible for maintaining business office systems Benchmark Reference(s):	40
	FACTOR #7 - INTERPERSONAL RELATIONSHIPS -- Difficult contacts with patients and families, coordinate billing procedures with other departments Benchmark Reference(s):	60
WORKING CONDITIONS	FACTOR #8 - WORK ENVIRONMENT -- Office Benchmark Reference(s):	5
	FACTOR #9 - HAZARDS -- Regular explanations of service Benchmark Reference(s):	15
EFFORT	FACTOR #10 - PERSONAL DEMANDS -- Regular stress to meet deadlines Benchmark Reference(s):	40

TOTAL POINT EVALUATION: 385

JOB DESCRIPTION

Job Title: Physical Therapist

Department: Rehabilitation

Primary Function: Treats disabilities due to injury or illness by the use of physical agents of heat, light, water, electricity and therapeutic exercise and massage as prescribed by physician, and evaluates patient progress.

Reports to (Title):

Supervises (Title):

Typical Duties:

Administers treatment programs by the use of active and passive exercise programs.

Administers diagnostic and prognostic muscle, nerve, joint and functional ability tests.

Uses therapeutic heat, light, electricity and bathing procedures to assist in patient rehabilitation.

Documents treatment and patient responses and/or progress.

Assist physicians in planning physicial rehabilitation programs.

Trains patients in the use and care of various supports such as wheelchairs, crutches, canes and prosthetic and orthopedic devises.

Prerequisites: Graduate of an accredited school of Physical Therapy and a current license from the State Board.

Working Conditions:

Job Title: Physical Therapist (Continued)

APPROVED:	REVIEWED AND RETAINED:
______________________ Supervisor	______________________ Supervisor
______________________ Date	______________________ Date
______________________ Department Head	______________________ Department Head
______________________ Date	______________________ Date

JOB TITLE: PHYSICAL THERAPIST DATE:

	BASIS OF EVALUATION	POINTS
SKILL	<u>FACTOR #1 - MENTAL DEVELOPMENT</u> -- Must have specialized knowledge and skills Benchmark Reference(s):	60
	<u>FACTOR #2 - WORK EXPERIENCE</u> -- Must know hospital policies, and have completed internship in lower level duties Benchmark Reference(s):	45
	<u>FACTOR #3 - JUDGMENT</u> -- Follows professional practice required to solve specific problems Benchmark Reference(s):	30
RESPONSIBILITY	<u>FACTOR #4 - ERRORS AND LOSSES</u> -- Considerable care required to apply treatments appropriately Benchmark Reference(s):	30
	<u>FACTOR #5 - RESOURCE UTILIZATION</u> -- Responsibility for utilization of major equipment Benchmark Reference(s):	30
	<u>FACTOR #6 - SYSTEMS AND DATA</u> -- Shares responsibility for the rehabilitation of a patient Benchmark Reference(s):	30
	<u>FACTOR #7 - INTERPERSONAL RELATIONSHIPS</u> -- Frequent and physical contact with patients Benchmark Reference(s):	30
WORKING CONDITIONS	<u>FACTOR #8 - WORK ENVIRONMENT</u> -- Regular exposure to disagreeable work elements Benchmark Reference(s):	15
	<u>FACTOR #9 - HAZARDS</u> -- Frequent strain manipulating patients Benchmark Reference(s):	15
EFFORT	<u>FACTOR #10 - PERSONAL DEMANDS</u> -- Constant standing, walking, with regular periods of lifting Benchmark Reference(s):	30

TOTAL POINT EVALUATION: 315

JOB DESCRIPTION

Job Title: Electroencephalograph Technician (EEG Technician)

Department: Technical Services

Primary Function: Measures impulse frequencies and differences in electrical potential of various areas of the brain to obtain data for use in diagnosing brain disorders by means of electroencephalograph (EEG).

Reports To (Title):

Supervises (Title):

Typical Duties:

Studies patient's medical record to obtain history and to identify potential symptoms during test.

Attaches electrodes and operates electroencephalograph, noting reactions and unusual wave characteristics.

Studies tracings during test and marks any evidence of disorders on graph.

Writes reports indicating unusual wave characteristics and communicates results to physician.

Prepares and assures patient regarding the nature of test.

Performs clerical duties to report and record test results.

Assists in maintaining inventory of department supplies and replenishing stock.

Maintains equipment in good operating condition.

Prerequisites: On-the-job training under the supervision of an experienced technician.

Working Conditions:

Job Title: Electroencephalograph Technician - EEG Technician (Continued)

APPROVED:	REVIEWED AND RETAINED:
Supervisor	Supervisor
Date	Date
Department Head	Department Head
Date	Date

JOB TITLE: ELECTROENCEPHALOGRAPH TECHNICIAN DATE:

	BASIS OF EVALUATION	POINTS
SKILL	FACTOR #1 - MENTAL DEVELOPMENT -- Requires basic knowledge of EKG testing Benchmark Reference(s):	30
	FACTOR #2 - WORK EXPERIENCE -- Basic on-the-job training required Benchmark Reference(s):	30
	FACTOR #3 - JUDGMENT -- Detailed job procedures, some room for judgment Benchmark Reference(s):	20
RESPONSIBILITY	FACTOR #4 - ERRORS AND LOSSES -- Normal care required to obtain accurate test results Benchmark Reference(s):	20
	FACTOR #5 - RESOURCE UTILIZATION -- Uses EEG machine Benchmark Reference(s):	20
	FACTOR #6 - SYSTEMS AND DATA -- Works as part of team Benchmark Reference(s):	20
	FACTOR #7 - INTERPERSONAL RELATIONSHIPS -- Contacts with patient Benchmark Reference(s):	30
WORKING CONDITIONS	FACTOR #8 - WORK ENVIRONMENT -- Limited exposure to disagreeable work elements Benchmark Reference(s):	10
	FACTOR #9 - HAZARDS -- Occasional minor abuse Benchmark Reference(s):	10
EFFORT	FACTOR #10 - PERSONAL DEMANDS -- Requires close attention for accurate results, frequent standing Benchmark Reference(s):	20

TOTAL POINT EVALUATION: 210

JOB DESCRIPTION

Job Title:	Electrocardiograph Technician (EKG Technician)
Department:	Technical Services
Primary Function:	Administers routine electrocardiograph (EKG) tests used in the diagnosis of heart ailments.
Reports To (Title):	
Supervises (Title):	
Typical Duties:	Analyzes patient's medical records to obtain information on the potential for unusual reaction or symptoms during test. Attaches electrodes and observes electrical output. Identifies sections of tracings which are unusual or noteworthy by pressing marker button and cuts and mounts tracings. Prepares and assures patient regarding nature of test. Instructs patient to perform physicial exercise if ordered by physician. Maintains equipment in good operating condition and reports significant defects. Performs clerical duties to report and record test results. Assists in maintaining inventory of supplies and replenishing stock. Communicates with patient's physician concerning results. May participate as a team member during cardiac arrest calls.
Prerequisites:	On-the-job training under the supervision of an experienced technician.

Job Title: Electrocardiograph Technician - EKG Technician (Continued)

Working Conditions:

APPROVED:	REVIEWED AND RETAINED:
______________________ Supervisor	______________________ Supervisor
______________________ Date	______________________ Date
______________________ Department Head	______________________ Department Head
______________________ Date	______________________ Date

JOB TITLE: ELECTROCARDIOGRAPH TECHNICIAN DATE:

	BASIS OF EVALUATION	POINTS
SKILL	FACTOR #1 - MENTAL DEVELOPMENT -- No specialized knowledge required Benchmark Reference(s):	15
	FACTOR #2 - WORK EXPERIENCE -- On-the-job training required Benchmark Reference(s):	30
	FACTOR #3 - JUDGMENT -- Detailed job procedures, some room for judgment Benchmark Reference(s):	20
RESPONSIBILITY	FACTOR #4 - ERRORS AND LOSSES -- Normal care required for accurate tests Benchmark Reference(s):	20
	FACTOR #5 - RESOURCE UTILIZATION -- Uses EKG machine Benchmark Reference(s):	20
	FACTOR #6 - SYSTEMS AND DATA -- Works as part of a team Benchmark Reference(s):	20
	FACTOR #7 - INTERPERSONAL RELATIONSHIPS -- Contacts with patient Benchmark Reference(s):	30
WORKING CONDITIONS	FACTOR #8 - WORK ENVIRONMENT -- Limited exposure to disagreeable work elements Benchmark Reference(s):	10
	FACTOR #9 - HAZARDS -- Occasional minor abuse Benchmark Reference(s):	10
EFFORT	FACTOR #10 - PERSONAL DEMANDS -- Close attention for accurate results Benchmark Reference(s):	20

TOTAL POINT EVALUATION: 195

JOB DESCRIPTION

Job Title: Respiratory Therapist (Certified)

Department: Technical Services

Primary Function: Sets up and operates various types of oxygen and inhalation equipment to administer medically approved gases, drugs, and therapeutic treatments to improve the cardiorespiratory functioning.

Reports To (Title):

Supervises (Title):

Typical Duties:

Reviews physicians' orders to verify prescription and order for treatment.

Obtains, sets up, operates, and regulates all types of respiratory therapy equipment.

Obtains and prepares medications according to prescription.

Administers IPPB and aerosal treatments.

Performs chest physiotherapy, postural drainage, incentive spirometry and basic pulmonary function tests.

Drains and analyzes arterial blood.

Charts patient information regarding treatment times, duration, therapy used, results, and general condition.

Instructs patient on treatment techniques and procedures to be performed to allay fears and anxieties.

Observes patient during therapy for any adverse reaction.

Disassembles, washes, sterilizes and reassembles equipment.

Maintains adequate supply of gases, medications, supplies, and equipment.

May serve as an integral member of cardiopulmonary resuscitation team and be responsible for the maintenance of emergency ventilation apparatus.

Job Title: Respiratory Therapist-Certified (Continued)

Prerequisites:

Working Conditions:

APPROVED:	REVIEWED AND RETAINED:
Supervisor	Supervisor
Date	Date
Department Head	Department Head
Date	Date

JOB TITLE: RESPIRATORY THERAPIST (CERTIFIED) DATE:

	BASIS OF EVALUATION	POINTS
SKILL	FACTOR #1 - MENTAL DEVELOPMENT -- Specific knowledge in a specialized field required Benchmark Reference(s):	45
SKILL	FACTOR #2 - WORK EXPERIENCE -- Must learn policies and procedures in the hospital Benchmark Reference(s):	45
SKILL	FACTOR #3 - JUDGMENT -- Follows standard practice, uses judgment from time to time Benchmark Reference(s):	30
RESPONSIBILITY	FACTOR #4 - ERRORS AND LOSSES -- Constant care to assure therapy properly and safely applied Benchmark Reference(s):	40
RESPONSIBILITY	FACTOR #5 - RESOURCE UTILIZATION -- Uses equipment and responsible for its maintenance Benchmark Reference(s):	20
RESPONSIBILITY	FACTOR #6 - SYSTEMS AND DATA -- Works as part of a team Benchmark Reference(s):	20
RESPONSIBILITY	FACTOR #7 - INTERPERSONAL RELATIONSHIPS -- Regular and substantive contacts with patients in all areas of the hospital Benchmark Reference(s):	45
WORKING CONDITIONS	FACTOR #8 - WORK ENVIRONMENT -- Regular exposure to disagreeable work elements Benchmark Reference(s):	15
WORKING CONDITIONS	FACTOR #9 - HAZARDS -- Exposure to infectious patients Benchmark Reference(s):	15
EFFORT	FACTOR #10 - PERSONAL DEMANDS -- Requires much standing and close care Benchmark Reference(s):	20

TOTAL POINT EVALUATION: 295

JOB DESCRIPTION

<u>Job Title</u>: Laundry and Linen Supervisor

<u>Department</u>: Laundry

<u>Primary Function</u>: Supervises, coordinates, and trains all laundry personnel for scheduled workload. Maintains production records and hours worked of personnel.

<u>Reports to (Title)</u>:

<u>Supervises (Title)</u>:

<u>Typical Duties</u>:

Inspects laundered articles to insure cleanliness and that proper methods are used.

Directs the requisition of replacement for worn linens.

Plans the changes, additions, and improvements to the laundry unit.

Reports needed repairs to the maintenance department.

Directs staff in the performing of sewing work and preparation of surgical packs.

Directs daily pick-up and delivery of laundry.

<u>Prerequisites</u>: Demonstrates a thorough knowledge of laundry procedures and practices of the hospital.

<u>Working Conditions</u>:

APPROVED:	REVIEWED AND RETAINED:
______________________	______________________
Supervisor	Supervisor
______________________	______________________
Date	Date
______________________	______________________
Department Head	Department Head
______________________	______________________
Date	Date

JOB TITLE: LAUNDRY AND LINEN SUPERVISOR DATE:

	BASIS OF EVALUATION	POINTS
SKILL	FACTOR #1 - MENTAL DEVELOPMENT -- General knowledge of all laundry procedures required Benchmark Reference(s):	30
	FACTOR #2 - WORK EXPERIENCE -- Must be proficient to train other laundry workers Benchmark Reference(s):	45
	FACTOR #3 - JUDGMENT -- Detailed procedures, some judgment Benchmark Reference(s):	20
RESPONSIBILITY	FACTOR #4 - ERRORS AND LOSSES -- Normal care required Benchmark Reference(s):	20
	FACTOR #5 - RESOURCE UTILIZATION -- Affects utilization of co-workers Benchmark Reference(s):	20
	FACTOR #6 - SYSTEMS AND DATA -- Team leader Benchmark Reference(s):	30
	FACTOR #7 - INTERPERSONAL RELATIONSHIPS -- Makes daily work assignments Benchmark Reference(s):	30
WORKING CONDITIONS	FACTOR #8 - WORK ENVIRONMENT -- Regular exposure to disagreeable work elements Benchmark Reference(s):	15
	FACTOR #9 - HAZARDS -- Some hazards Benchmark Reference(s):	10
EFFORT	FACTOR #10 - PERSONAL DEMANDS -- Close attention to assure process running smoothly Benchmark Reference(s):	20

TOTAL POINT EVALUATION: 240

JOB DESCRIPTION

Job Title: Washer

Department: Laundry

Primary Function: Collects, separates and washes dirty linens from all areas of the hospital in such a way as to prevent cross contamination.

Reports to (Title):

Supervises (Title):

Typical Duties: Collects dirty linen from all departments and nursing units.

Separates and sorts the different types of linens.

Weighs and records weight being processed.

Loads and unloads washers.

Separates and performs prescribed procedures for contaminated linens.

Measures proper amount of chemicals for each washload.

Prerequisites: None

Working Conditions:

APPROVED:

____
Supervisor

____
Date

____
Department Head

____
Date

REVIEWED AND RETAINED:

____
Supervisor

____
Date

____
Department Head

____
Date

JOB TITLE: WASHER DATE:

	BASIS OF EVALUATION	POINTS
SKILL	FACTOR #1 - MENTAL DEVELOPMENT -- No specialized knowledge required Benchmark Reference(s):	15
	FACTOR #2 - WORK EXPERIENCE -- On-the-job indoctrination to learn machines Benchmark Reference(s):	15
	FACTOR #3 - JUDGMENT -- Simple routine work Benchmark Reference(s):	10
RESPONSIBILITY	FACTOR #4 - ERRORS AND LOSSES -- Minor responsibility for errors Benchmark Reference(s):	10
	FACTOR #5 - RESOURCE UTILIZATION -- Limited resource utilization Benchmark Reference(s):	10
	FACTOR #6 - SYSTEMS AND DATA -- Limited responsibility for systems and data Benchmark Reference(s):	10
	FACTOR #7 - INTERPERSONAL RELATIONSHIPS -- Assists other washers Benchmark Reference(s):	15
WORKING CONDITIONS	FACTOR #8 - WORK ENVIRONMENT -- Continuous exposure to disagreeable work elements Benchmark Reference(s):	20
	FACTOR #9 - HAZARDS -- Some contact with contaminated linen, carries heavy loads of laundry, moving machinery Benchmark Reference(s):	15
EFFORT	FACTOR #10 - PERSONAL DEMANDS -- Regular lifting Benchmark Reference(s):	30

TOTAL POINT EVALUATION: 150

JOB DESCRIPTION

Job Title: Medical Records Clerk

Department: Medical Records

Primary Function: Provides clerical support in the medical record handling processes and assists in compiling data for statistical reports.

Reports to (Title):

Supervises (Title):

Typical Duties: Reviews medical records of discharged patients for their completeness.

Assembles records into established order for permanent filing.

Records deficiencies and maintains follow-up until records are complete and received.

Checks daily census report and corrects errors.

Answers telephone and provides information if appropriate.

Records diagnoses and operations on specified forms.

Assists in other medical record processing such as filing and retrieval of medical records.

Prerequisites: Knowledge of alpha/numeric filing procedures. No prior experience required.

Working Conditions:

Job Title: Medical Records Clerk (Continued)

APPROVED:	REVIEWED AND RETAINED:
______________________	______________________
Supervisor	Supervisor
______________________	______________________
Date	Date
______________________	______________________
Department Head	Department Head
______________________	______________________
Date	Date

JOB TITLE: MEDICAL RECORDS CLERK DATE:

	BASIS OF EVALUATION	POINTS
SKILL	FACTOR #1 - MENTAL DEVELOPMENT -- No specialized knowledge required Benchmark Reference(s):	15
	FACTOR #2 - WORK EXPERIENCE -- Must learn some medical terminology and proper sequence of medical records Benchmark Reference(s):	30
	FACTOR #3 - JUDGMENT -- Detailed job procedures, some follow-up responsibility Benchmark Reference(s):	20
RESPONSIBILITY	FACTOR #4 - ERRORS AND LOSSES -- Normal care required to assure accurate, complete records Benchmark Reference(s):	20
	FACTOR #5 - RESOURCE UTILIZATION -- Controls reports (census) etc., which has impact on hospital finances Benchmark Reference(s):	20
	FACTOR #6 - SYSTEMS AND DATA -- Handles confidential information Benchmark Reference(s):	20
	FACTOR #7 - INTERPERSONAL RELATIONSHIPS -- Assists other medical records clerks Benchmark Reference(s):	15
WORKING CONDITIONS	FACTOR #8 - WORK ENVIRONMENT -- Office conditions Benchmark Reference(s):	5
	FACTOR #9 - HAZARDS -- Normal office routine Benchmark Reference(s):	5
EFFORT	FACTOR #10 - PERSONAL DEMANDS -- Normal work place attention Benchmark Reference(s):	10

TOTAL POINT EVALUATION: 160

JOB DESCRIPTION

Job Title: Medical Records Technician, ART

Department: Medical Records

Primary Function: Assists in the supervision of the medical records office and participates in record handling and processing.

Reports to (Title):

Supervises (Title):

Typical Duties: Compiles medical record statistical reports such as birth and death records, utilization, occupancy rates and outpatient services.

Participates in coding diseases and operations according to established procedures and maintains indexes.

Assists medical staff in locating information and conducting records research.

Responds to requests for medical information on patients' charts and answers departmental correspondence.

Assists in training, hiring and evaluation of department personnel.

Reviews records for accuracy and completeness according to hospital standards.

May represent the hospital in court involving subpoena of medical records.

Prerequisites: Completion of an accredited course in medical records and successful completion on an examination.

Working Conditions:

Job Title: Medical Records Technician, ART (Continued)

APPROVED:	REVIEWED AND RETAINED:
Supervisor	Supervisor
Date	Date
Department Head	Department Head
Date	Date

JOB TITLE: MEDICAL RECORDS TECHNICIAN ART DATE:

	BASIS OF EVALUATION	POINTS
SKILL	FACTOR #1 - MENTAL DEVELOPMENT-- Must understand legal requirements of recordkeeping, a specialized occupational field Benchmark Reference(s):	45
SKILL	FACTOR #2 - WORK EXPERIENCE -- Proficiency in clerical positions, where to locate information Benchmark Reference(s):	45
SKILL	FACTOR #3 - JUDGMENT -- Follows standard practice, makes decision to release information Benchmark Reference(s):	30
RESPONSIBILITY	FACTOR #4 - ERRORS AND LOSSES -- Requires considerable care to assure records kept accurately and legally Benchmark Reference(s):	30
RESPONSIBILITY	FACTOR #5 - RESOURCE UTILIZATION -- Directs activities of other clerks Benchmark Reference(s):	30
RESPONSIBILITY	FACTOR #6 - SYSTEMS AND DATA -- Shares responsibilities for recordkeeping process, regularly handles confidential information Benchmark Reference(s):	30
RESPONSIBILITY	FACTOR #7 - INTERPERSONAL RELATIONSHIPS -- Deals with requests regarding medical information from doctors, public financial institutions Benchmark Reference(s):	45
WORKING CONDITIONS	FACTOR #8 - WORK ENVIRONMENT -- Pleasant environment Benchmark Reference(s):	5
WORKING CONDITIONS	FACTOR #9 - HAZARDS -- Normal office routine Benchmark Reference(s):	5
EFFORT	FACTOR #10 - PERSONAL DEMANDS -- Close attention to be sure medical records are in proper order Benchmark Reference(s):	20

TOTAL POINT EVALUATION: 285

JOB DESCRIPTION

Job Title: Medical Transcriptionist

Department: Medical Records

Primary Function: Transcribes medical reports for inclusion in patient medical record, for transmission to physicians and for other medical care facilities.

Reports to (Title):

Supervises (Title):

Typical Duties:

Transcribes medical reports on diagnostic workups, operative procedures and summaries for inclusion in medical records.

Proofreads and verifies work performed.

Keeps records of work performed.

Answers staff requests for dictation.

Types various medical reports and records from handwritten or rough copy.

Uses dictionaries, text references and other reference materials as required to assure accurate medical documentation.

Prerequisites: Graduation from a vocational training program for medical transcriptionists.

Working Conditions:

APPROVED:	REVIEWED AND RETAINED:
______________________	______________________
Supervisor	Supervisor
______________________	______________________
Date	Date
______________________	______________________
Department Head	Department Head
______________________	______________________
Date	Date

JOB TITLE: MEDICAL TRANSCRIPTIONIST DATE:

	BASIS OF EVALUATION	POINTS
SKILL	FACTOR #1 - MENTAL DEVELOPMENT -- Must use dictaphone and have knowledge of medical terminology Benchmark Reference(s):	45
	FACTOR #2 - WORK EXPERIENCE -- Must learn to operate in-house equipment and procedures Benchmark Reference(s):	30
	FACTOR #3 - JUDGMENT -- Uses standard practice to format, etc., must interpret physicians on tapes Benchmark Reference(s):	30
RESPONSIBILITY	FACTOR #4 - ERRORS AND LOSSES -- Considerable care to assure accurate documents Benchmark Reference(s):	30
	FACTOR #5 - RESOURCE UTILIZATION -- Uses office machines Benchmark Reference(s):	20
	FACTOR #6 - SYSTEMS AND DATA -- Works as part of team, regularly handles confidential information Benchmark Reference(s):	30
	FACTOR #7 - INTERPERSONAL RELATIONSHIPS -- Little contact with other departments Benchmark Reference(s):	15
WORKING CONDITIONS	FACTOR #8 - WORK ENVIRONMENT -- Required to remain at work station Benchmark Reference(s):	10
	FACTOR #9 - HAZARDS -- Normal office routine Benchmark Reference(s):	5
EFFORT	FACTOR #10 - PERSONAL DEMANDS -- Requires continuous concentration for transcribing, must proofread Benchmark Reference(s):	30

TOTAL POINT EVALUATION: 245

JOB DESCRIPTION

Job Title: Personnel Assistant

Department: Personnel

Primary Function: Performs a wide variety of support activities including employment interviewing for hourly and clerical jobs, recordkeeping, assisting with benefits and other personnel services.

Reports to (Title):

Supervises (Title):

Typical Duties: Interviews and prescreens applicants for hourly and clerical positions.

Checks references on employment applications as required.

Processes benefit forms for sending to insurance carrier, assuring that all forms are properly completed and the necessary forms attached.

Explains insurance coverage and procedures to employees as requested.

Prepares and updates job positions.

Keeps up-to-date files of training and development materials.

Keeps personnel files culled and up-to-date.

Types reports, correspondence and other materials.

Maintains records on absenteeism, turnover, overtime, etc.

Prerequisites: Demonstrates basic clerical skills. Previous experience in dealing with the public.

Working Conditions:

Job Title: Personnel Assistant (Continued)

APPROVED:	REVIEWED AND RETAINED:
Supervisor	Supervisor
Date	Date
Department Head	Department Head
Date	Date

JOB TITLE: PERSONNEL ASSISTANT DATE:

	BASIS OF EVALUATION	POINTS
SKILL	FACTOR #1 - MENTAL DEVELOPMENT -- Requires general knowledge of personnel policies and procedures Benchmark Reference(s):	30
	FACTOR #2 - WORK EXPERIENCE -- Must have a thorough knowledge of personnel policies, benefits and recordkeeping Benchmark Reference(s):	45
	FACTOR #3 - JUDGMENT -- Quotes and interprets hospital policy, uses standard practice Benchmark Reference(s):	30
RESPONSIBILITY	FACTOR #4 - ERRORS AND LOSSES -- Requires considerable care to accurately interpret policies to employees Benchmark Reference(s):	30
	FACTOR #5 - RESOURCE UTILIZATION -- Uses office machines, distributes training materials Benchmark Reference(s):	20
	FACTOR #6 - SYSTEMS AND DATA -- Shares responsibility for recruiting and proper processing of personnel records Benchmark Reference(s):	30
	FACTOR #7 - INTERPERSONAL RELATIONSHIPS -- Interacts with managers and supervisors from all areas of the hospital and new applicants Benchmark Reference(s):	45
WORKING CONDITIONS	FACTOR #8 - WORK ENVIRONMENT -- Office conditions Benchmark Reference(s):	5
	FACTOR #9 - HAZARDS -- Normal office routine Benchmark Reference(s):	5
EFFORT	FACTOR #10 - PERSONAL DEMANDS -- Close attention to assure accurate personnel records Benchmark Reference(s):	20
	TOTAL POINT EVALUATION:	260

V. Summary of Evaluations

POSITION EVALUATION WORKSHEET

POINT FACTOR RATING

RADIOLOGY POSITION	MENTAL DEVELOPMENT	WORK EXPERIENCE	JUDGMENT	ERRORS AND LOSSES	RESOURCE UTILIZATION	SYSTEMS AND DATA	INTERPERSONAL RELATIONSHIPS	WORK ENVIRONMENT	HAZARDS	PERSONAL DEMANDS	TOTAL
Chief Radiologic Technologist	60	75	40	40	40	50	60	10	20	30	425
Radiologic Technologist R.T.	45	30	30	30	20	30	45	10	20	20	280

POSITION EVALUATION WORKSHEET

POINT FACTOR RATING

CLINICAL LABORATORY POSITION	MENTAL DEVELOPMENT	WORK EXPERIENCE	JUDGMENT	ERRORS AND LOSSES	RESOURCE UTILIZATION	SYSTEMS AND DATA	INTERPERSONAL RELATIONSHIPS	WORK ENVIRONMENT	HAZARDS	PERSONAL DEMANDS	TOTAL
Chief Laboratory Technologist	75	75	40	40	40	50	60	10	15	30	435
Medical Laboratory Technician M.L.T.	30	30	30	40	20	30	30	15	20	20	265
Medical Technologist (MTASCP)	45	45	30	40	30	30	30	15	20	30	315
Laboratory Supervisor (Section)	60	60	30	40	30	40	45	15	20	30	370
Laboratory Aide	15	15	10	10	10	20	15	15	20	10	140

POSITION EVALUATION WORKSHEET

POINT FACTOR RATING

CENTRAL SERVICE POSITION	MENTAL DEVELOPMENT	WORK EXPERIENCE	JUDGMENT	ERRORS AND LOSSES	RESOURCE UTILIZATION	SYSTEMS AND DATA	INTERPERSONAL RELATIONSHIPS	WORK ENVIRONMENT	HAZARDS	PERSONAL DEMANDS	TOTAL
Central Service Technician	15	30	10	20	20	20	15	15	20	30	195

POSITION EVALUATION WORKSHEET

POINT FACTOR RATING

NURSING SERVICE POSITION	MENTAL DEVELOPMENT	WORK EXPERIENCE	JUDGMENT	ERRORS AND LOSSES	RESOURCE UTILIZATION	SYSTEMS AND DATA	INTERPERSONAL RELATIONSHIPS	WORK ENVIRONMENT	HAZARDS	PERSONAL DEMANDS	TOTAL
Staff Nurse	45	45	30	40	30	40	45	15	15	20	325
Instructor Staff Develop-ment	60	60	40	40	30	40	75	10	10	20	385
Nursing Assistant	15	30	20	20	10	20	15	15	15	30	190
Nursing Supervisor	60	60	40	50	50	50	60	10	15	30	425
Unit Clerk/ Unit Secre-tary	30	30	20	20	20	30	30	10	10	20	220
Infection Control Nurse	60	45	30	40	30	40	45	10	10	20	330
Licensed Practical Nurse	30	30	20	30	20	30	30	15	15	30	250
Department Secretary	45	45	30	20	20	30	30	5	5	20	250
Head Nurse	60	60	40	40	40	40	60	15	15	30	400

POSITION EVALUATION WORKSHEET

POINT FACTOR RATING

NURSING SERVICE POSITION	MENTAL DEVELOPMENT	WORK EXPERIENCE	JUDGMENT	ERRORS AND LOSSES	RESOURCE UTILIZATION	SYSTEMS AND DATA	INTERPERSONAL RELATIONSHIPS	WORK ENVIRONMENT	HAZARDS	PERSONAL DEMANDS	TOTAL
Assistant Director	60	75	40	40	50	50	75	10	15	30	445

POSITION EVALUATION WORKSHEET

POINT FACTOR RATING

DIETETICS POSITION	MENTAL DEVELOPMENT	WORK EXPERIENCE	JUDGMENT	ERRORS AND LOSSES	RESOURCE UTILIZATION	SYSTEMS AND DATA	INTERPERSONAL RELATIONSHIPS	WORK ENVIRONMENT	HAZARDS	PERSONAL DEMANDS	TOTAL
Dietary Tray Handler	15	15	10	20	10	20	15	15	15	20	155
First Cook	45	45	20	20	30	30	30	20	15	30	285
Staff Dietitian	60	45	40	30	30	30	60	10	10	20	335
Food Service Director	60	60	40	40	40	40	60	10	10	30	390
Dietary Clerk	15	30	20	20	20	20	15	10	5	20	175

POSITION EVALUATION WORKSHEET

POINT FACTOR RATING

HOUSEKEEPING POSITION	MENTAL DEVELOPMENT	WORK EXPERIENCE	JUDGMENT	ERRORS AND LOSSES	RESOURCE UTILIZATION	SYSTEMS AND DATA	INTERPERSONAL RELATIONSHIPS	WORK ENVIRONMENT	HAZARDS	PERSONAL DEMANDS	TOTAL
Executive Housekeeper	45	60	40	30	40	40	45	10	15	30	355
Housekeeping Aide	15	15	10	10	10	20	15	15	15	30	155
Housekeeping Supervisor	30	45	20	20	20	30	30	15	10	20	240

POSITION EVALUATION WORKSHEET

POINT FACTOR RATING

PLANT ENGINEERING POSITION	MENTAL DEVELOPMENT	WORK EXPERIENCE	JUDGMENT	ERRORS AND LOSSES	RESOURCE UTILIZATION	SYSTEMS AND DATA	INTERPERSONAL RELATIONSHIPS	WORK ENVIRONMENT	HAZARDS	PERSONAL DEMANDS	TOTAL
Security Guard	15	30	30	20	20	20	30	10	10	20	205
Maintenance Mechanic	30	45	30	30	20	20	30	20	15	30	270
Maintenance Supervisor	45	60	30	30	30	30	45	15	10	20	315
Plant Operations Manager	60	75	40	50	50	50	60	10	10	30	435

POSITION EVALUATION WORKSHEET

POINT FACTOR RATING

PURCHASING POSITION	MENTAL DEVELOPMENT	WORK EXPERIENCE	JUDGMENT	ERRORS AND LOSSES	RESOURCE UTILIZATION	SYSTEMS AND DATA	INTERPERSONAL RELATIONSHIPS	WORK ENVIRONMENT	HAZARDS	PERSONAL DEMANDS	TOTAL
Purchasing Agent	45	45	30	30	30	30	45	5	10	20	290

POSITION EVALUATION WORKSHEET

POINT FACTOR RATING

FINANCIAL MANAGEMENT POSITION	MENTAL DEVELOPMENT	WORK EXPERIENCE	JUDGMENT	ERRORS AND LOSSES	RESOURCE UTILIZATION	SYSTEMS AND DATA	INTERPERSONAL RELATIONSHIPS	WORK ENVIRONMENT	HAZARDS	PERSONAL DEMANDS	TOTAL
PBX/Switchboard Operator	15	30	20	20	10	20	30	10	10	10	175
Payroll Clerk	30	45	20	30	30	30	30	5	10	20	250
Admitting Clerk	15	30	20	20	20	20	45	10	10	20	210
Admitting Supervisor	45	45	30	30	30	40	45	5	15	20	305
Insurance Billing Clerk	30	30	30	30	20	20	30	5	5	20	220
Accountant	60	45	30	40	30	40	45	5	10	30	335
Business Office Supervisor	45	60	40	40	40	40	60	5	15	40	385

POSITION EVALUATION WORKSHEET

POINT FACTOR RATING

REHABILITATION POSITION	MENTAL DEVELOPMENT	WORK EXPERIENCE	JUDGMENT	ERRORS AND LOSSES	RESOURCE UTILIZATION	SYSTEMS AND DATA	INTERPERSONAL RELATIONSHIPS	WORK ENVIRONMENT	HAZARDS	PERSONAL DEMANDS	TOTAL
Physical Therapist	60	45	30	30	30	30	30	15	15	30	315

POSITION EVALUATION WORKSHEET

POINT FACTOR RATING

TECHNICAL SERVICES POSITION	MENTAL DEVELOPMENT	WORK EXPERIENCE	JUDGMENT	ERRORS AND LOSSES	RESOURCE UTILIZATION	SYSTEMS AND DATA	INTERPERSONAL RELATIONSHIPS	WORK ENVIRONMENT	HAZARDS	PERSONAL DEMANDS	TOTAL
EEG Technician	30	30	20	20	20	20	30	10	10	20	210
EKG Technician	15	30	20	20	20	20	30	10	10	20	195
Respiratory Therapist	45	45	30	40	20	20	45	15	15	20	295

POSITION EVALUATION WORKSHEET

POINT FACTOR RATING

LAUNDRY POSITION	MENTAL DEVELOPMENT	WORK EXPERIENCE	JUDGMENT	ERRORS AND LOSSES	RESOURCE UTILIZATION	SYSTEMS AND DATA	INTERPERSONAL RELATIONSHIPS	WORK ENVIRONMENT	HAZARDS	PERSONAL DEMANDS	TOTAL
Laundry and Linen Supervisor	30	45	20	20	20	30	30	15	10	20	240
Washer	15	15	10	10	10	10	15	20	15	30	150

POSITION EVALUATION WORKSHEET

POINT FACTOR RATING

MEDICAL RECORDS POSITION	MENTAL DEVELOPMENT	WORK EXPERIENCE	JUDGMENT	ERRORS AND LOSSES	RESOURCE UTILIZATION	SYSTEMS AND DATA	INTERPERSONAL RELATIONSHIPS	WORK ENVIRONMENT	HAZARDS	PERSONAL DEMANDS	TOTAL
Medical Records Clerk	15	30	20	20	20	20	15	5	5	10	160
Medical Records Technician A.R.T.	45	45	30	30	30	30	45	5	5	20	285
Medical Transcription-ist	45	30	30	30	20	30	15	10	5	30	245

POSITION EVALUATION WORKSHEET

POINT FACTOR RATING

PERSONNEL / POSITION	MENTAL DEVELOPMENT	WORK EXPERIENCE	JUDGMENT	ERRORS AND LOSSES	RESOURCE UTILIZATION	SYSTEMS AND DATA	INTERPERSONAL RELATIONSHIPS	WORK ENVIRONMENT	HAZARDS	PERSONAL DEMANDS	TOTAL
Personnel Assistant	30	45	30	30	20	30	45	5	5	20	260

VI. Evaluation Results of Generic Positions

EVALUATION RESULTS OF GENERIC POSITIONS

	PTS.	GRADE
ASSISTANT DIRECTOR, NURSING SERVICE	445	22
CHIEF LABORATORY TECHNOLOGIST	435	21
PLANT OPERATIONS MANAGER	435	21
CHIEF RADIOLOGIC TECHNOLOGIST	425	21
NURSING SUPERVISOR	425	21
HEAD NURSE	400	20
FOOD SERVICE DIRECTOR	390	20
INSTRUCTOR, STAFF DEVELOPMENT	385	20
BUSINESS OFFICE SUPERVISOR	385	20
LABORATORY SUPERVISOR (SECTION)	370	19
EXECUTIVE HOUSEKEEPER	355	19
ACCOUNTANT	335	18
STAFF DIETITIAN	335	18
INFECTION CONTROL NURSE	330	18
STAFF NURSE	325	18
PHYSICAL THERAPIST	315	18
MAINTENANCE SUPERVISOR	315	18
MEDICAL TECHNOLOGIST	315	18
ADMITTING SUPERVISOR	305	17
RESPIRATORY THERAPIST (CERTIFIED)	295	17
PURCHASING AGENT	290	17

	PTS.	GRADE
FIRST COOK	285	17
MEDICAL RECORDS TECHNICIAN, ART	285	17
RADIOLOGIC TECHNOLOGIST	280	17
MAINTENANCE MECHANIC	270	16
MEDICAL LABORATORY TECHNICIAN	265	16
PERSONNEL ASSISTANT	260	16
LICENSED PRACTICAL NURSE	250	15
DEPT. SECRETARY, NURSING SERVICE	250	15
PAYROLL CLERK	250	15
MEDICAL TRANSCRIPTIONIST	245	15
LAUNDRY AND LINEN SUPERVISOR	240	15
HOUSEKEEPING SUPERVISOR	240	15
UNIT CLERK/UNIT SECRETARY	220	14
INSURANCE BILLING CLERK	220	14
EEG TECHNICIAN	210	14
ADMITTING CLERK	210	14
SECURITY GUARD	205	13
EKG TECHNICIAN	195	13
CENTRAL SERVICE TECHNICIAN	195	13
NURSING ASSISTANT	190	13
PBX/SWITCHBOARD OPERATOR	175	12
DIETARY CLERK	175	12
MEDICAL RECORDS CLERK	160	12

	PTS.	GRADE
HOUSEKEEPING AIDE	155	11
DIETARY TRAY HANDLER (DIETARY AIDE)	155	11
WASHER	150	11
LABORATORY AIDE	140	11

APPENDIX B: INCENTIVE COMPENSATION PLAN UNDER PROSPECTIVE PRICING

From the hospital's perspective, DRG prospective pricing creates dual management challenges: managing productivity and managing "volumes"-- that is, managing service utilization.*

Under cost-based reimbursement, the more services provided, the more the hospital received, up to some limit. Under prospective pricing, the relationship between a hospital's cost and Medicare revenues is severed; the hospital will now be at risk for the difference between its costs and the prices set and paid per discharge by Medicare.

To manage volume, hospitals must work especially with physicians, to control length of stay and the use of ancillary services for acute patient care. Managing productivity, of course, means controlling the unit cost of individual services, which includes labor costs.

DRG Impact on Labor Cost

The DRG approach emphasizes hospital output, thus heightening the awareness of hospital inputs, especially labor input. As a result, human resources management is rising significantly as an important issue. Productivity, defined as the output that can be produced from a given input, will be a key component as will the management of related personnel expenses. Improved productivity will be the key to success under DRGs. The prospective pricing system provides incentives for hospitals to save rather than spend, as was characterized by the cost-based retrospective payment system.

Labor cost is a major line item, making up over one-half of total hospital expenditures for most institutions. In addition, labor

*For more detailed information on DRGs read DRGs: A Practitioner's Guide, Paul L. Grimaldi and Julie A. Micheletti, Pluribus Press, Inc., 160 E. Illinois, Chicago, IL.

cost tends to be easier to adjust in the short run than fixed costs of buildings and equipment. Hospitals under prospective pricing will attempt to cut their labor costs by reducing staff, by finding ways to make existing staff more productive, by resisting pressure to increase wages, by changing staffing patterns and skill-mix, and by using incentives in ways that will result in more efficient operations.

Incentives

A recent IRS ruling says that nonprofit hospitals may now establish profit sharing or incentive compensation plans based on net surplus. The ruling specifically states that it is necessary for health care institutions to be profitable and that it is perfectly proper for those responsible to be rewarded accordingly.

An effective compensation program is one that attracts qualified employees, retains them, provides internal equity, recognizes superior performance, and enhances the motivation of hospital personnel through total systems incentives.

The use of incentive programs to favorably affect the quality and quantity of employee productivity has been an accepted practice in American industrial and service enterprises and the proprietary health care sector.

A monetary return for increased productivity, as a result of either group or individual effort to exceed a predetermined productivity norm or standard, is not incompatible with the nonprofit character of health care institutions.

The main purpose of productivity-oriented employee incentive programs should be to reduce an institution's operating costs to the lowest level, while maintaining high-quality patient care.

Rewarding employees for increased effort and initiative is

appropriate, and may take the form of periodic monetary or deferred payments.

Under prospective pricing, managers probably will have to redesign their jobs, and adapt programs and techniques once thought to be outside their scope of non-profit health care functions. What is needed are incentives that:

1. Cut vertically through the organization and strengthen organizational bonds;
2. Focus on the qualitative aspects of work-- on new ideas and more effective teamwork;
3. Appeal not only to the financial needs but also to social ego fulfillment needs of employees;
4. Facilitate change, the introduction of new techniques, processes, equipment and services; and
5. Relate people to the common goal of improving organizational effectiveness.

Types of Incentive Plans

Two major categories of incentive plans are emerging-- discretionary and target performance plans. In discretionary plans, the award may not be related to specific, predetermined achievements. Rather the award is based on the collective decision of a compensation committee which has reviewed the overall performance.

Target performance plans are based on specific predetermined achievements and the amount of awards related to specific achievment levels. Either type of plan may be developed for individual group rewards. Group rewards can be important as part of a team-building effort, but ultimately the achievers prefer rewards based on individual accomplishments.

Regardless of the type of incentive plan, the achievement target or overall performance should be based upon the hospital's objectives. Individual group or department targets identified for incentive awards should be geared to the strategic organizational goals.

Factors to be Considered

Incentive systems require careful consideration of such factors as the basis upon which such payments are calculated, the negative attitudinal problems toward compensation, and the implementation and administration of the incentive plan.

The basis of payment is a question that is always raised when incentives are discussed among nonprofit health care professionals. In the industrial sector and the proprietary health care sector, there are a variety of incentive plans. These range from relatively simple discretionary plans to highly complex performance-based plans in which payment is received on immediate cash payouts, deferred compensation, and stock and equity opportunities. The majority of plans, however, regardless of simplicity or complexity, relate payment to some form of quantifiable performance measurements. For example, in the industrial sector, incentive compensation may be based on specific goals in the following areas: profit to sales ratio, return on investment, cost reduction targets, inventory to shipments ratio, or fixed assets to shipment ratios. Some may have no application in the nonprofit health care sector, especially in states where the amount of surplus that can be earned may be restricted by legislative direction. In the proprietary health care sector, incentive awards are an important aspect of the compensation plan.

Basing incentive compensation entirely on achieving profit or surplus goals may be questionable regardless of statutory limits on such accumulation. This does not preclude basing incentive compensation on other factors such as implementing specific cost reductions, increasing revenue in specific areas, meeting marketing goals, and increasing efficiency or productivity.

The negative attitude of health care professionals toward incentive compensation is another factor that must be addressed and overcome.

How to Start

One should begin with a feasibility study among the board and key executive groups, assessing attitudes and the current objective-setting process within the institution. Such a study should help determine if the environment is conducive to implementing an incentive compensation plan.

The ultimate responsiblity for an incentive system rests with the trustees. No plan should be implemented without board approval. An intensive educational program for both trustees and employees should be part of the incentive compensation plan.

The executive compensation committee of the board should assume the following responsibilities in administering the plan:

* determine eligibility for participation in the plan
* establish the fund, and
* determine the method and basis of payment

Of course, the chief executive officer will usually delegate duties for implementing the plan.

An incentive plan should be added to the individual compensation plan. Keep in mind that it is not a substitute for a competitive base salary. An incentive compensation plan rewards achievements beyond normal expectations. It is not a method of increasing gross compensation or circumventing an established salary-increase policy. The award plans are not guaranteed, the amount will vary annually, depending on the individual's performance and the institution's financial condition. Awards should be substantial enough to be meaningful. Specific objectives upon which incentives will be based must be known in advance and agreed upon by participants.

The health care sector team needs a standard as a goal, and it needs to be rewarded when the goal is exceeded. Incentive compensation is one method for rewarding outstanding performance that is now getting the attention it deserves in the health field.

APPENDIX C: GLOSSARY OF COMPENSATION TERMS AND DEFINITIONS

GLOSSARY OF COMPENSATION TERMS AND DEFINITIONS

The majority of the following definitions were compiled from the book entitled Dictionary of Personnel Management and Labor Relations by Jay M. Shafritz, published in 1980 by Moore Publishing Company, Inc., Oak Park, IL.

Benchmark - any standard that is identified with sufficient detail so that other similar classifications can be compared as being above, below, or comparable to the "benchmark" standard.

Compensation Program - the facet of management concerned with the selection, development, and direction of the programs that implement an organization's financial reward system.

Competitive Wages - rates of pay that an employer, in competition with other employers, must offer if he or she is to recruit and retain employees.

Comp-Ratio (C/R) - the relationship (compensation ratio) of current actual salary to the jobs structure midpoint of the salary range.

Demotion - transfer to a job in a lower grade.

Exempt Employee - an employee whose job is assigned a grade on the annual structure.

External Equity - a measure of an employee's wages when the compensation for his or her position is compared to the labor market as a whole within a region, profession, or industry.

Going Rate - a rate most commonly paid to workers in a given occupation for a specific locale.

Grade - an established level or zone of difficulty. Positions of the same difficulty and responsibility tend to be placed in the same grade even though the content of the work differs greatly.

Internal Equity - a measure of an employee's wages when the compensation for his or her position is compared to similar positions within the same organization.

Job Analysis - the determination of a position's specific tasks and of the knowledge, skills, and abilities that an incumbent should possess.

Job Content - the duties and responsibilities of a specific position.

Job Description - a summary of the duties and responsibilities of a job.

Job Evaluation - a process that attempts to determine the relative worth of a position. It emphasizes a formal comparison of the duties and responsibilities in order to ascertain the worth, rank, or classification of one position relative to all others in an organization.

Job Grading - a method of comparing jobs on a "whole job" basis in order to rank such jobs in a hierarchy from highest to lowest.

Job Rate - usually expressed as the range midpoint and represents the going rate for a fully qualified, experienced employee who is performing satisfactorily.

Job Sharing - two people, each working part-time, sharing the same job.

Lateral Transfer - a transfer to a job in the same grade.

Longevity Pay - salary additions based on length of service.

Maximum Job Rate - the maximum pay level for a job assigned to that range.

Merit Adjustment - an increase an employee receives in recognition of performance.

Merit Guidelines - the policy and procedures that relate pay to performance.

Merit Increase - a raise in pay based upon a favorable review of an employee's performance.

Merit Programs - a set of procedures designed to reward employees with salary increases reflecting their on-the-job performance.

Minimum Job Rate - represents the salary normally paid to a new employee without any applicable job experience, who meets the minimum qualifications for the position.

Non-Exempt - an employee whose job is assigned a grade on the hourly structure.

Organization Structure - the arrangement of an organization into divisions, departments, and units according to a specific criteria.

Performance Appraisal - a formal method by which an organization documents the work performance of its employees.

Point System (also called the Point Method) - the most widely used method of job evaluation, in which the relative worth of the jobs being evaluated is determined by totaling the number of points assigned to the various factors applicable to each of the jobs.

Productivity - measured relationship between the quantity (and quality) of results produced and the quantity of resources required for production. Productivity is, in essence, a measure of the work efficiency of an individual, a work unit, or a whole organization.

Promotion - a transfer to a job in a higher grade.

Range Maximum - the highest wage rate established in a labor grade.

Range Minimum - the lowest wage rate established in a labor grade.

Range Spread - the distance between the lowest wage rate and highest wage rate in a labor grade.

Salary Compression - the shrinking difference in pay given to newcomers as opposed to the amount paid to experienced regulars.

Salary Range - the range of hourly, weekly, biweekly, semimonthly, monthly, or annual rates applicable to a job grade, usually expressed by a minimum job rate and maximum job rate.

Salary Review Date - the date on which an employee becomes eligible for a salary adjustment. In most situations this is the anniversary of the date of hire.

Salary Structure - a uniform system used for the organization wages paid to an employee.

Shift Differential - the extra compensation paid as an inducement to accept shift work outside of "normal daytime business hours."

Structural Adjustment - changes in the salary structure.

REFERENCES

1. AHA Special Report #3, Medicare Prospective Pricing: Legislative Summary and Management Implications, American Hospital Association, Chicago, April, 1983.

2. Browdy, Jerold D., Health Care Executive Compensation: Principles and Strategies, Aspen Systems Corp., Rockville, MD. 1983.

3. Grimaldi, Paul L. and Micheletti, Julie A., DRG Update: Medicare's Prospective Payment Plan, Pluribus Press, Inc., Chicago, 1983.

4. Grimaldi, Paul L. and Micheletti, Julie A., DRGs: A Practitioner's Guide, Pluribus Press, Inc., Chicago, 1983.

5. Grover, Pat N., Cost Containment Through Employee Incentives Program, Aspen Systems Corp., Rockville, MD, 1977.

6. Managing Under Medicare Prospective Pricing, American Hospital Association, Chicago, Oct., 1983.

7. Metzger, Bert L., Enhancing the Motivating of Hospital Personnel Through Total Systems Incentives, Profit Sharing Research Foundation, Evanston, IL 1967.

8. Shakno, Robert, Physician's Guide to DRGs, Pluribus Press Inc., Chicago, 1984.